Doctors and Patients

Doctors and Patients

Doctors
and
Patients

What We Feel About You

Peter H. Berczeller, M.D.

A LISA DREW BOOK

MACMILLAN PUBLISHING COMPANY
NEW YORK

MAXWELL MACMILLAN CANADA
TORONTO

MAXWELL MACMILLAN INTERNATIONAL
NEW YORK   OXFORD   SINGAPORE   SYDNEY

A Lisa Drew Book
Macmillan Publishing Company
866 Third Avenue
New York, NY 10022

Maxwell Macmillan Canada, Inc.
1200 Eglinton Avenue East
Suite 200
Don Mills, Ontario M3C 3N1

Macmillan Publishing Company is part of the Maxwell
Communication Group of Companies.

Library of Congress Cataloging-in-Publication Data
Berczeller, Peter H.
Doctors and patients: what we feel about you / Peter H. Berczeller
p. cm.
"A Lisa Drew book."
ISBN 978-1-9821-0228-9
1. Physician and patient. 2. Physicians—Attitudes.
I. Title.
R727.3.B46 1994
610.69′6—dc20   93-23991

Macmillan books are available at special discounts for bulk purchases
for sales promotions, premiums, fund-raising, or educational use. For
details, contact: Special Sales Director, Macmillan Publishing
Company, 866 Third Avenue, New York, NY 10022

Book design by Ellen R. Sasahara

10 9 8 7 6 5 4 3 2 1

Printed in the United States of America

To Adrienne, who saved my life, and continues to do it every day.

To my father, who first showed me what it means to be a doctor.

*To my patients, every one of them, who taught me how to be
a physician.*

Acknowledgments

My thanks go to my editor, Lisa Drew, who believed in this book and whose interest during its creation was as effective as any bedside manner I have ever seen during my many years in medicine.

The cooperation and helpfulness of her assistant, Katherine Boyle, my telephone and fax pal, was limitless, and I appreciate her concern immensely.

Charles Grodin, in an act of completely spontaneous kindness, introduced me to Lisa Drew and thus deserves some of the credit (or responsibility, depending on how you look at it) for the publication of this book.

Ira Berkow, the longtime literary adviser to the aspiring writers of my family, has my deep gratitude for his generosity on so many levels.

Marian Saunders, my assistant and dear friend, deserves special thanks for her great devotion to our patients as well as to my personal welfare.

My mother, Marie Berczeller, has always had confidence in me, and I hope that this book will live up to her expectations.

My son Paul, a writer, in whose literary judgment I have great faith, provided me with many valuable insights during the creation of this book.

John, my actor son, contributed his artistic sensibilities during the same time, and I am lovingly grateful to him.

My foster son, Nick Restifo, generously shared with me a younger doctor's views of some of the subjects I discussed in this book.

Acknowledgments

Lastly, my thanks go to David Friedman. I can only say to him what the man said who, without provocation, slapped the face of a Hungarian hitherto unknown to him: "You know what that's for!"

Contents

Preface

It is unfair but nevertheless it's true: we know much more about our patients than they know about us. The old-time docs, who made up in humanity what they lacked in knowledge, possessed a great deal of information about those under their care, and this was so especially because they also treated their families and often visited their homes. Nowadays the pendulum is swinging back, and the idea of treating the whole patient—his occupation, love life, and family problems included—has again become popular within the medical profession.

The public is understandably curious about what we doctors are really like behind our "professional" exterior. Yet I think that this curiosity mainly confines itself to questions about how we live, the looks of our wives, or, for that matter, how faithful we are to them. The answers to these questions, though, even if they are completely reliable, do nothing but satisfy idle speculation. Instead, we can do much, much better, because it is within our power to reveal something vastly more important, and that is the range and complexity of the feelings that we have toward our patients and toward what we do. In return, then, if these revelations could make patients understand that we have fears and conflicts just as they do, they might, we hope, see us more as thinking *and* feeling people, rather than as impersonal technicians.

Most doctors who see patients on a regular basis gain an insight into the anxiety and feelings of helplessness that disease brings about. Patients cope with these feelings in various ways, among them by their excessive dependency or unduly aggressive behavior. The experienced physician has learned to recognize these and other responses as symptoms and can more than occasionally relieve them if he can get the patient to "open up," to translate his emotions into words. The thought of serious illness, of something being wrong with the body, that motor whose smooth running is taken for granted, can be devastating. As an example, most patients are frightened by changes in laboratory values, even though they are not sure whether they are of real significance or not. What's more, as they are put through the assembly line from CAT scan to MRI to ultrasound, they look at the technician's face in the vain hope that a smile means that everything is all right. In other words, they are puzzled by the diagnostic process, yet they cling to any reassuring word while imagining the worst.

This is, of course, where the doctor comes in. I say "of course" because it is clear that the patient needs a guide to lead him through the unfamiliar terrain he is so reluctantly traversing. But the patient needs much more than a guide. He needs a lawyer, a scientist, a priest, and a best friend all rolled into one. In short, he desperately needs someone who, in a setting of warm personal contact, can help him make the most critical decisions of his life.

In the past, a patient's health and well-being depended mainly on the knowledge and experience of the doctor. With nothing much else to go on, since laboratory and x-ray procedures did not nearly have the importance they do today, it was reasonable for patients to invest doctors with mythical powers. They questioned very little, if anything at all, and certainly not why the doctor advised this or that. What's more, his caring was more or less taken for granted in a time of day and night house calls and relatively low fees. At the same time, his behavior, whether gruff or tender, or both, was accepted as one would accept that of an occasionally irritable but basically loving relative.

These days, though, patients act very differently toward us, and they routinely question our knowledge and judgment, rather than take anything for granted. In addition, some patients misinterpret it as a sign of our weakness that we require frequent help from laboratory tests, x-rays, and other physicians. The reality is very different. Good patient care is often a cooperative effort, and this search for assistance is a sign of our conscientiousness and commitment.

It is only natural that, if patients have gained insight into the way we take care of them and into how inexact a science medicine really is, they will also question our motivation, our degree of caring, and how important they really are to us—not as "cases" but as human beings. This uncertainty about us seems to be a favorite topic of conversation not only in waiting rooms but also on talk shows, and has captured a lot of attention in the popular literature.

We doctors are usually silent when these concerns come up. It seems forever that we have been unwilling to expose our deep feelings about patients and about illness, the two overpowering landmarks on our particular horizon. So the world is completely justified in judging us only by our behavior, since we keep the feelings that lead to the behavior so tightly under wraps.

This reluctance to "go public" has usually been explained away, rather glibly, by our expressions of fear of doing harm to patients if they ever gained insight into how we feel. In other words, we are afraid to even verbalize the *suggestion* that we are capable of having feelings of dislike for those who have entrusted us with their health and their lives, or, for instance, that we harbor some sexual thoughts about them. What's more, as another example, we are terribly reluctant to reveal that even we supposed experts in illness are as afraid of it as our patients.

So we have gone on, another silent minority, complaining only to each other about how unjustly we are treated by the very people we spend our lives trying to help.

Even to ourselves, and certainly to the rest of humanity, these emotions are a vast, unexplored area. I do not remember that, during my training or my years in practice, I even once had an in-depth conversation on this subject with other doctors. But then, do soldiers in battle speak out about their feelings about war? Instead, they will bitch about the cold food or the cruelty of the top sergeant, just as those in medical training argue about days off or the excessive number of patients under their care.

In day-to-day medicine, philosophizing is frowned upon, not the least because it takes time away from what is usually a frantic job. But there is also a macho side to this profession. The doctor is capable of seeing himself as someone apart, not completely answerable to the rules of the "civilians." Since when does the legendary cowboy reveal how he feels about himself, or the ranch, or roping cattle?

This book has only one purpose, although I admit that it is a large one, and that is to report the view from the inside. I believe that it is the appropriate time for me to do this after eight years of training and thirty-two years of private practice and teaching. It is also high time that the outside world be made aware of the complex feelings we have toward our patients as well as about disease, which in turn serves to both separate and unite us.

We touch each other on many levels. We deal with each other in the worst of times. We sometimes struggle over power or fight about money. We grapple with unwanted sexual feelings, and sometimes we fire the patient or he fires us. Illness is not funny, but interchanges with patients can be. Doctors live for that occasional glorious moment when they know what it is to win, when the diagnosis suddenly becomes clear, or when the patient dramatically improves. And they also dread that sudden turn in the patient's condition when it becomes obvious that the game is lost and that the patient will die.

Patients do resent doctors, and frequently for good reason. After seeing thousands of patients and getting along very well with most of them, I still wish that some of my exchanges with them had turned out differently. From my viewpoint now, I should sometimes have been less brusque, more understanding, less impatient. What's worse, we have among us our crooks, alcoholics, sexual molesters, and drug abusers, who, in the process of harming themselves, cause their innocent patients to suffer as well. In addition, we have any number of practitioners who are truly remote and who just don't care. It is a difficult thing to accept the presence of all these physicians in a profession that is known for its problem-solving qualities, when they themselves turn out to be the biggest problem.

Yet, based upon my lifelong impressions as the son and nephew of doctors, as a student, resident, practitioner, and teacher, I believe that most doctors mean well. It is true that most of us are not geniuses, but then, most of what we do does not demand that quality of us. Certainly we make plenty of mistakes. We suffer grievously when we become aware of them, and most of us consider it the equivalent of a mortal sin not to learn from them.

What's more, it is all too often too difficult to communicate with us, in person or on the telephone. Our hospital visits are probably too short, and we thoughtlessly don't warm a cold stethoscope before applying it to the chest. We delegate too little or too much authority to our office managers, so obtaining an appointment for the care of even an acute illness can be almost as distressing as being sick in the first place. The list of frustrations connected with doctors' ways and the environment that they create is, if not endless, certainly a long one.

And yet, patients and their families are not blameless, either. I have already mentioned how fear and feelings of helplessness bring about the kind of behavior most patients do not exhibit when they are well. Although most doctors understand very well that these are really symptoms, they can and do become angry and resentful because of the acting out on the part of the patient. But how are they to express this anger? They can't "tell the patient off" because that might worsen his condition. So they smolder, becoming either less sympathetic and somewhat remote or expressing excessive concern. Both extremes have the same significance, though, and that is that the doctor feels a conflict between his obligation to the patient and his resentment about the way he is being treated.

Families, under the guise of "my relative is sick, therefore I can act in any way I want to," sometimes harass doctors with threats of suit, repeated hostility, and the playing off of one physician against another. The doctor, who already has his hands full in dealing with the patient's medical problem, is thus forced to fight on two fronts. The relatives may have perfectly reasonable objections to the way the case is being managed, but their aggressive approach to the doctor does not make them equal players. They are, rather, snipers who cannot or will not engage in a constructive dialogue with the doctor based on a common purpose: "Let's get our patient better!"

I am well aware that a book cannot by itself change long-standing behavior and attitudes that are based on fear of the unknown, suspiciousness, differences in social class, and so on. I am convinced, though, that it is absolutely essential that patients finally gain insight into how we physicians feel about what we do, about illness, and about them in particular. Patients cannot do without us in a world that has not conquered, and probably will never conquer, disease. At the same time, we cannot do without them, either. I would like to think that a greater understanding of who we are will help to open up a true dialogue between partners, so that the ever more sophisticated and life-enhancing medicine being practiced today is not held back by distrust, suspicion, and ill feeling.

1

Quitting

DURING ALL MY YEARS in medicine, I always thought of retirement as something that happened to other doctors, to the "old guys." Usually the word applied to somebody who, before disappearing altogether, was seen in the hospital less and less often, and about whom one began to forget a little bit in the daily scheme of things. For instance, I am reminded of someone, let us call him Morris Bergman, whom no one ever called anything but Moe. He was a tall, thin, white-haired, red-faced man with a very loud voice who always wore a vest with his suit, invariably either a dark or light blue worsted, summer and winter. When I first met him, approximately thirty years ago, he did most of his talking in the doctors' coatroom and was already, according to him, "semiretired." He had never married and lived with his sister, who ceremoniously conveyed him to the main hospital entrance, daily, in an enormous fifties-vintage Chrysler. He would then make straight for the coat-room, and it was well known that if he captured you, it would take at least thirty or forty minutes to escape from his mono-logue of rambling reminiscences. His sister—for the coatroom also served her as a forum—avidly filled in all the details in his stories. When he finally left to "make rounds," she would seam-lessly continue the story that her brother had begun. Sadly, though, Moe would return from his rounds within no more than ten to fifteen minutes and it was evident that they had probably comprised no more than one patient. His sister would then hand the conversational baton back to him as the next wave of potential listeners filed into the coatroom.

It was hard to imagine that Moe had ever been like us, that he had ever been in the mainstream of the life of the hospital and considered by his colleagues to be much more than the relic he now was. Certainly the residents, ever sensitive to the nuances of change in status of their elders, underlined his increasing isolation by the unusually courteous way in which they behaved toward him. This was in marked contrast to the barely civil approach those of us in the supposedly respected group were accustomed to.

It is so difficult for someone in his early thirties, as I was then, to conceive of a time when the good times will have gone. What had happened to Moe was not at all unusual. He had been busy until his mid-sixties, and then his practice began to decline. He tried to rationalize it in his coatroom orations: "What can I do? The patients who started out with me years ago are now dying in bunches! I don't see any new patients because the young ones all go to young doctors!" After this, as usual, he threatened to retire "if the patients don't straighten out."

I sympathized with him each time we spoke, and falsely reassured him that my own practice had recently also been "not so good." After each of our conversations, I promised myself that, in contrast to him, I would get out before I was forced out. I would do anything rather than be in Moe's shoes thirty or forty years from then.

This was, of course, the bravado of a young man with very little experience. I did not take into account the reluctance of older people to part with something infinitely dear to them: the work that has sustained them throughout their adult lives. At the same time, I was not aware of how painful it is for doctors, however diminished, to forgo their "perks." When I say this,

2

though, I am not speaking of a significant income or special parking privileges but, rather, of the responsiveness that doctors elicit in other people. For instance, we cannot ever kick the habit of being the center of attention, just like a quarterback, when we get into a huddle with a patient's family. It is just as impossible to replace the burning facial sensation (in a young girl it would be called a blush) that accompanies praise or gratitude or appreciation or whatever it is called that indicates to the doctor that the patient feels that he has come through for him.

As matters turned out, my resolve was never tested. I did not phase out gradually, and when I made my decision to leave practice I was still very much in demand. In a sense, this more dramatic exit made my leave-taking from my patients that much harder. Neither they nor I had had enough warning or time to make saying good-bye any easier.

There were two transitions in the past that were very painful for me. The first was the changeover, after graduation from medical school, from student to intern. Although it was infinitely satisfying to see the "M.D." after my name (I remember frequent glances at my new checkbook during the first few days after graduation), I constantly reminded myself of the large gaps in my knowledge and the many possible clinical situations where these gaps could easily become embarrassingly apparent. I soon realized that the hospital hierarchy had the same reservations about an intern's capabilities that I had, and it took me several years (as it is supposed to) to gain trust in my own abilities.

But at the end of my training, when I switched roles again, from elder statesman trainee to rookie practitioner, my hard-won self-confidence was again threatened. This time I was not so much concerned about my knowledge or my capability of competently handling a variety of problems. I was very concerned, however, not only about where my first private patient would come from (a common worry, by the way, for people in my situation) but also why someone would wish to pay *me* for my services when there were so many more experienced and better doctors available. Probably to counteract these doubts, I went into a frenzy of activity. I let it be known that I was available for referrals from my hospital's emergency room twenty-four hours a day, and I made house calls for older doctors, so that, ever so slowly, it seemed to me, a few patients a week began to trickle into my infrequently used office.

But despite the fact that my practice was growing, I still felt like a student. That is, I acted and thought according to the lessons I had learned in my training, and because of this, I considered each encounter with a patient to be a test of my knowledge. If things went well, I thought that it was because I had learned the lesson well. If things went poorly, it signified that it was my fault and that the lesson had escaped me.

I was on a constant roller coaster of emotion, going from relief to guilt and back again several times a day. When the phone rang at night, as it did frequently, I was ever ready to assume the worst—in other words, that I was being called about someone who had "gone bad" because of some error on my part.

This went on for a few years, but my inner turmoil, if anything, stimulated the growth of my practice. I was known as conscientious, as someone who "left no stone unturned," qualities that attracted referrals from patients as well as from other doctors. But I was also tense and self-conscious and I derived very little pleasure from what I was doing.

What I was missing, I see in retrospect, was the larger view. I did not understand that there is much more to medicine than what are really reflex mechanical activities such as diagnosing and treating, which are part of what is called "managing a case." I did not yet understand that patients care much more about prognosis—that is, what is ultimately going to happen to them—than about diagnosis, the definition of what is wrong.

4

In my drive for perfection, I focused all my efforts on understanding disease, something that in turn left very little room for understanding, and not just listening to, the concerns of patients.

I cannot say that my failings became clear to me at any particular moment and that this dramatic revelation changed my approach. It was rather that, a few years after my frenetic beginnings, I began to notice a subtle but increasing ease in dealing with my day-to-day activities, so that I began to feel less "tested" every time I looked at a patient. In looking back, I do not believe that the quality of my care changed significantly at this point, but it seems to me that my pleasure in providing the care certainly did.

This change in outlook culminated, a few years later, in a feeling that I have had until now and that will never leave me: I love medicine! This is an intense emotion that I share with many of my colleagues, but it is one that we are reluctant to admit to anyone but ourselves. The reason for this hesitation is our justifiable concern that patients may well resent our loving something that represents only suffering to them.

This feeling is not only that I like what I do but also that medicine is so much a part of my life that I would not feel whole without it. Of course, I respect the science that is its basis, just as I respect the technology that allows us to be only slightly less blind in our perennial pursuit (we never do quite catch up) of disease. But respect is a cool emotion, while love is irrational, and it is exactly the irrational aspect of medicine that makes us love it so. What any one body will do at any one time is completely unpredictable, and this is the flip side of the predictability of science. Solutions based on common sense frequently come out better than those that were intricately calculated. We are exhilarated by living on the edge, by facing situations that test the very outer limits of our capabilities. We also gain a rare insight into other peoples' lives, and if we are both skillful and fortunate, we have warm and memorable contact with a whole cross section of humanity.

In addition, some of the reasons why we love are as unknowable as the answers to questions such as how we love and how much we love. *Whether* we love medicine, on the other hand, is never in doubt. What else can it be than love if we think about the object all day long, dream about it at night, and are terribly jealous of anyone who has a closer relationship to it than we do? What's more, isn't it love if this passion never leaves us, however much age has finally made passive spectators of us all?

My latest transition, though, in which I quit (I prefer this word to *retire* because it has a more voluntary ring for me) private practice, touched me much more deeply than the two changes of which I have already spoken. Early in a medical career, it is expected that people and places will be left behind as the trainee advances on a well-laid-out path. Anxiety, frustration, and insecurity are the unavoidable baggage one carries along, even though they, as in my case, often stimulate achievement. But to leave terribly familiar territory, which I had run, and paced, and stumbled over for more than thirty years, was a wrench for which I was not and could not have been prepared. It was not a vast territory, but it was mine. It contained my office and my staff, with whom I regularly spent more hours per day than I did with my family. Most important, it contained my patients. Without them, of course, neither office nor staff nor I would have had any kind of function.

Quitting—or retiring, if you will—is far-reaching but still just a decision. Saying good-bye, on the other hand, is the dark side of this conspiracy with yourself. In this case at least, and in contrast to the usual moralistic warning, first you pay and *then* you play.

I said good-bye in every way I could. I wrote a letter to each of my active patients, and I personally communicated with as many of them as I could. Some of them in turn answered me or sent me presents, which prompted me to respond one more time.

Happily, something funny happened from time to time that helped to break the gloomy farewell mood. Lisl Hilfling, a long-time patient in her late eighties, had been companion and secretary to a famous Austrian opera singer for over forty years and still goes to the opera at least once a week. Except for mild arthritis, she is remarkably healthy and has no evidence of senility. I fully expect her to live to the age of one hundred, barring some unforeseen accident. Whenever Lisl visited my office over the years, she never failed to complain bitterly about my lack of interest in her well-being, my total lack of success in dealing with her joint pains, and the generally poor way in which my office was run. What's more, she had a host of friends who were also my patients. When these ladies came to see me, they felt compelled to describe to me—at great length and in confidence, of course—the extent of Lisl's unhappiness with my care.

The obvious question, which I frequently asked her, was why, given the extent of her discontent, she continued to be my patient. The reply was always vague, so that my feelings toward her remained permanently fixed in an uncomfortable limbo somewhere between her dissatisfaction and my medical responsibility.

Lisl called me as soon as she received my announcement. She was evidently crying and told me how irreplaceable I would be and how very much she would miss me in the future. I was amazed. I could not reconcile her sorrow with her previous behavior, and I told her so. She answered, evidently surprised by my lack of insight: "That was then. But now it's serious!"

Despite these all-too-few comic interludes, my patients and I rapidly came to understand that our bonds were being broken and that this had to be the end. When people who love each other separate, there is always the hope, expressed or unexpressed, that they will see each other again. But my patients and I had to part for good despite our intimate and warm relationship because their medical care had always been the one driving force behind our connection. If I was no longer providing this care, then it was essential for them to take up with someone new as soon as possible, so that there would be no loss of continuity.

What I just said is what I believe, and that is the way it should be. Yet the less rational part of myself wanted to hold on at whatever cost. I did not really want to let these people go, despite the fact that I no longer could be responsible for their day-to-day welfare. Was it egotism that pushed me into *having* to retain that sense of power over others that comes so naturally with our work? Or was it, despite the fact that it was I who initiated the breakup, a fear of being abandoned by hundreds of people at the same time, people who had believed in me?

I cannot pinpoint the reason for my wistfulness, my reluctance to let go. Whatever the cause of this terminal cowardice on my part, the last, best thing I could do for my patients was to make the clean break.

Then there was the problem of leaving my colleagues. Could it all really be over with so quickly that I was already so enmeshed in nostalgia? The medical way of life lends itself so readily to brooding about the past. I am forever ruminating about the thousands of encounters, like atomic collisions, that happened between me and those I taught (or who taught me) and those I helped (or who helped me) in taking care of patients. I remember discussions about hoarse voices, and breaths that smelled like nail polish remover, and yellow skin. We argued about whether there was fluid in the abdomen or whether the patient was just fat, about whether the spleen was enlarged or whether it was just muscle that we were feeling. I remember the medical equivalent of a coffee table book with a warm dedication and signed "gratefully" by my six third-year students of a particular year (do not ask me which one). On the other hand, I will never forget that sensation, on many more than one occasion, of being the absolute village idiot when a patient died suddenly for no apparent reason after an illness that had resisted diagnosis. Afterward we sat there, the residents and I, in those gloomy, poorly ventilated, artificially lit conference rooms, with the stunned look of witnesses to a tragic accident. As relatives often do, we wanted to deny what had happened, wanted the truth to go away. For the next hour or two, or however long it took us to verbalize the initial shock, there was a sense of communion among us. Age and rank differences melted away for the moment as even the youngest and most inexperienced of us—the third-year student, for example—had to realize that this particular case had been, flat out, beyond all our capabilities.

I also remember the peculiar shorthand that is used between doctors who work together a lot. When my favorite surgeon, Steve, would half-yell to me from one end of the cafeteria to the other, "His temperature's down, but she's still bleeding," I found out exactly what I needed to know about the two patients who worried me most on that particular day. I had confidence in his judgment and he in mine, and what's more, we knew each other too well to go into niceties or greetings.

I will always feel and think like a doctor; that part of me can never be erased. But the mutual understanding built on trust and nurtured by time that I enjoyed over the years with so many looms large and can never be replaced.

*　*　*

A career in medicine does not run full circle. Rather, it evolves in a line that, although it meanders at times, can still be recognized for what it is. In our never-ending need to make sense of what has happened to us (with the added titillation that there may be *no* sense in it at all), it is more than an exercise in nostalgia to capture both the beginning and the end for our memory. These two extreme points of the one line define in their own way how it was going to be, and how it was, although it is never clear exactly when the influence of the beginning is supplanted by the anticipation of the end.

For several weeks after I stopped seeing patients, I was the medical equivalent of a lame duck. I filled out forms, completed charts, and generally went through the completely unfamiliar routine of winding down. For the first time in many years, I had large amounts of time to dispose of, something that made me vastly more uncomfortable than my usual time pressures. I arrived in the office late and left early, exactly what I had always criticized in the "nine-to-five doctors," and I ambled down the street nowadays. I continued to sit in my consultation room and completely neglected my good old standbys, the examining rooms. I put off the packing of the mementos of all those years, the "Best Dad" statuette, family pictures, diplomas, little notes written to me by my children when they were very young. I looked at the ancient dust on the seldom-cleaned venetian blinds that had taken on the status of lava, it was so thick and so dark. And I took a farewell glance at the ancient, paper-stuffed, drafty window embrasures that I counted as mementos as well, the only ones to stay when every other vestige of my long presence here would be gone.

I also thought of symmetry, how things had started and how they were ending. I remembered the visit of my first office patient ever and how embarrassed I had been. He was a writer for the *New York Times*, in his fifties, and he complained of pain in his stomach. Naturally, I had to examine his abdomen, but my examining table had not yet been delivered. While I was taking his history, I felt more and more agitated. Where in the world could he lie down so I could properly check him for tenderness or even a mass? I realized very soon that I was looking at the only sizable flat surface, besides the floor, in my office. I asked him to loosen his trousers, cleared my desk, and asked him to lie down on it. Fortunately, he was not tall, and just about fit. While I was examining him, I nervously chattered on about battlefield conditions, how untold numbers of healthy babies had been delivered on kitchen tables, and the like. I don't know what he must have been thinking, but I can imagine: "Agitated doctor, too eager to please; underequipped office. How do I get out of here?"

Happily, I found nothing wrong, makeshift arrangements or not. I wrote out a prescription on the multipurpose desk and asked him to call me in a few days. Needless to say, I never heard from him again.

I must have hoped, unconsciously, that there would be some symbolic significance, some signpost to the future, in the very last patient visit before my leaving. As often happens with high expectations, the reality fell flat. Nothing much transpired in my interview with Frank. Medically it was straightforward: a routine visit for follow-up of high blood pressure and a renewal of prescriptions. Our personal relationship had always been, as they say, correct, but never effusive. When I told him of my decision, he accepted the news with equanimity. I made sure that he had adequate follow-up, and that was it.

I don't know what I had expected. I felt deflated, cheated. At least my first patient had been memorable, if only because of the comedy of errors connected with his visit. But if I was searching for symmetry, for an end-of-the-line cathartic experience, for an unforgettable farewell performance by both the patient and myself, I had clearly not found it.

Of course I would, many times in the future, think back to

some of the thousands of incidents that together made up the body of my work over all those years. Next to these, one encounter, even if its timing is crucial, should not assume undue significance. But the last experience in a series of many is precious. And if it has a meaning of its own in addition, and not just its lastness to distinguish it, then it is unique and should be savored for as long as memory holds out against the infiltration of time.

As it happened, Frank was only the last *official* patient to be seen. By that I mean that he had an appointment, my findings were duly noted in the chart, and he paid me for the visit. My house call on Brina a few days later, though, marked the real end of my activities.

She was a lady in her early eighties, and her hair was always dyed jet-black and arranged in a beehive. I had been her doctor for at least fifteen years, and during all that time she had been relatively well except for slightly elevated blood pressure and occasional severe tension headaches. In recent times, I had found a cancer of the rectum, and this had spread, causing her to be jaundiced. Each time she came to the office she was thinner, and in the weeks immediately before I quit, I did not hear from her at all. I had always kept a mental checklist of those patients who were in real trouble and somehow got in touch with them if their silence was unduly long. Brina certainly belonged high up on this list. While ruminating one day in my soon-to-be-dismantled headquarters, and in a burst of self-pity identifying intensely with Napoleon in Elba (or maybe even Saint Helena), the checklist alarm buzzed within my head and I called her. The nurse who attended her at home answered and told me that Brina was quite incoherent and too weak to come to the telephone under any circumstances.

I felt relieved that Brina was still alive. In view of her very poor outlook, this was selfish of me. But I knew that I would have felt very guilty if she had died before I saw her one more time. The upheaval in my own life might thus accidentally have been responsible for an irreversible break in communications between us.

I told the nurse to tell Brina that I was coming immediately, and on the way to her house I thought about how little I knew of the way she lived. With patients scattered all over the metropolitan area, my mobility hampered by the dense Manhattan traffic but my conscience somewhat eased by my seeing patients in emergency rooms who would normally have been seen at home, I had stopped making regular house calls years ago. At the same time, though, I felt guilty because I had never stopped believing that seeing a patient in his own environment adds immeasurably to what the doctor, if he wants to do a really good job, should know about him.

That is not to say that I did not, very occasionally, make a home visit. It was always a special circumstance, though: a fellow doctor, someone who lived around the corner from my office, or a ninety-seven-year-old man whom I had known since I was ten. With these rare exceptions, and especially in recent years, like many of my colleagues I played a sort of Russian roulette when faced with a sick patient calling from home. The reason I use this term, which is admittedly not usually associated with medical matters, is that when a decision is made over the telephone in this kind of situation, things can easily blow up in your face at any time from there on in. The temptation is strong for a busy doctor to treat without seeing the patient when the situation does not *sound* critical. Yet I have learned to be very, very cautious about exactly who can be handled in this way: generally only established patients with trivial new complaints or the same group with old complaints that have been adequately investigated previously. Just one call in a medical lifetime from a policeman reporting the death of someone thought "not sick enough to come in" is more than enough to justify this extreme caution.

Can an emergency room visit be equated to a doctor's visit at home? No, not really. Speaking strictly medically, there is no comparison. The availability of the hospital's laboratory and x-ray facilities, as well as its consultants, is a major advantage to the emergency room patient. That is, if he is very sick. But if he comes there with, for example, flulike symptoms or diarrhea, complaints that used to bring a visit from the faithful family practitioner, the emergency room visit will not only not make him better but might make him feel worse. Waiting for hours in a drafty hallway, only to be seen by a harried doctor he has never seen before and who is obliged to order expensive blood tests and x-rays just not to "miss" anything is hardly the way to treat a patient's mild illness. On the contrary, this is a time to be babied, to stay in a warm bed, and to be reassured by a friendly presence. And certainly when the patient is beyond help and requires only a familiar environment rather than the senseless commuting to an impersonal hospital "facility," home is the place to be.

In our many encounters, Brina had always been well dressed, well mannered, and her conversation reflected her appearance. The apartment, not surprisingly, fit in perfectly with my previous impressions. She was sitting on a couch that had been made up as a bed. Several bookcases lined the walls of the large one-room studio. The titles of the books on the shelves and the prints in rather ornate frames pointed to their owner as someone who, maybe up to ten years ago, had made a conscious effort to keep up with culture as she saw it.

As we say in medicine, her affect was blunted. That is, although she seemed to recognize me, she did not show any surprise at my sudden appearance nor did she attempt to make conversation with me. She was dressed in a vaguely Oriental dressing gown, her black hair was, as usual, in perfect order, and she was even thinner than I had remembered. I told her immediately that I was there as a friend rather than as a doctor.

Since long-ingrained habits die hard, however, and since I am famously poor at small talk, I found myself asking the same questions that I had usually asked patients in my other life, which had ended so recently. I inquired about her appetite, if she was able to sleep, and whether she was in pain. She answered slowly, and in a low voice, that she didn't need anything. I could not think of anything else to say. There was no need to tell her of the change that had taken place in my life because, under any circumstance, this was the last time we would ever see each other. We sat there quietly, and I noticed that we had begun to hold hands. Brina and I were even. She asked nothing of me, and since she was obviously terminal (I have always hated that ominous word), I was no longer under any obligation to try to get her to respond to desperate life-prolonging maneuvers.

Going out was a term used in the fifties and sixties instead of *dying*. To borrow a phrase from that time, in early August 1992 Brina was going out of her life. At the same time, her doctor was going out of his career. Isn't that symmetry?

2

Who's in Charge Here?

PEOPLE OFTEN SAY IT straight to a doctor's face: "I don't like [or "I hate"] doctors." The tone is sometimes embarrassed, and "present company excluded" is added for the sake of politeness, but there is no question about it, it is a genuine feeling that is being expressed. But can we take it at face value? I don't really think so, although I have no doubt that some doctors are hateful, having met quite a few of them myself. Yet this statement is heard so often and in so many different settings that it is obvious that it has a deeper, a more universal, meaning.

We are all terribly frightened by illness and by death. Doesn't it give a patient a sense of some control, then, if, instead of having to face the bottomless void of the inevitable, he can express negative feelings against the doctor, who is at least another human being and not just one of nature's random punishments?

What's more, all of us patients are conflicted. On the one hand, we sense deep down that we must obey the doctor, lest we not get better; and the fantasy that is attached is that the doctor can make us even worse if he is made angry by any insubordination on our part. On the other hand, we resent having to share, or give up altogether, decision-making powers in matters related to our life and health, the only really significant things we own. In addition, we are wary of being too dependent on a stranger who, for all we know, may, whatever he claims, not even be doing the right thing to keep us afloat.

But doctors are also very conflicted. Our expectation is that all patients will give us immediate obedience and respect—and 100 percent of the time at that! But how do we justify such a notion, which appears pretty arrogant, at least on the surface? We keep telling ourselves that it is because we have studied so hard and have so painstakingly acquired our training and experience that we expect this unquestioning acceptance of our edicts. And besides, if we have sacrificed so much of our time and energy for the ultimate sake of our patients, should we not at least be rewarded by their keeping quiet and doing what we tell them to do?

Yet the reality is totally different. Anyone who hopes to practice medicine with any degree of effectiveness has to come to grips with the fact that patients very definitely have a mind of their own. This does not mean, of course, that, much of the time, patients do not follow the doctor's advice. When they "comply," though, I am convinced that they do so because they have made a conscious decision to go along with us and not because they have been intimidated by our brilliance or by our status. Still, most doctors, for reasons of professional and personal self-esteem, prefer to look at patient compliance as something that is due them, rather than something that is earned. In the long run, though, *why* patient and doctor agree is much less important than the fact that they do, something that can only be of benefit to the patient.

"Resistant" patients, although much smaller in number, take up a disproportionate amount of the doctor's time and energy. These are the patients who either reject out of hand most or all that the doctor has to offer, or who achieve the same purpose by negotiating the subject to death. These individuals most often have very little insight into what they are doing, and truly believe that their behavior is due to the "right to know everything" or to "have control over my own destiny." What happens frequently, of course, is that these patients go from doctor to doctor and are never satisfied, because they expect help on the one hand but reserve for themselves the privilege of setting all the rules on the other.

We doctors as a group are emotionally rather insecure. Whether we start out this way or whether the unstable and unpredictable nature of what we do makes us this way is not clear. Yet because of this insecurity and tendency to guilt, any negative reaction on the part of the patient is immediately interpreted by us not only as lack of respect for our professional opinion but also as an aggressive act toward us personally.

The physician knows he can't express his anger openly because he is afraid of worsening the patient's condition. Patients do not want to be disapproved of by their doctors, whatever their own behavior. A man with angina may well have an episode of chest pain after his doctor has spoken to him brusquely, for example, just as a woman with a tendency to migraines may have a severe headache in the same situation. So the physician learns that he has to control his own behavior very strictly, sometimes to the point of throwing up his hands and letting the patient do what he wants. He is so frustrated that he wishes the patient would go away and bother another doctor for a change, but he cannot get himself to actually "fire" him. Once in a while, the patient leaves on his own. The good times are brief, though, because there is always another resistant patient just around the corner!

Somebody who alternates between being compliant and resistant is even more difficult to deal with than the individual who is resistant all the time. Just when the doctor is lulled into a sense of security by the apparently full cooperation of the patient, there is a complete turnaround. For no obvious reason, the benign acceptance of the doctor's advice is replaced by disagreement with his handling of virtually every aspect of the case. Ultimately this black cloud also disappears, and peace and harmony again reign; for how long, nobody knows.

Early in my career, Han Ming Wong was referred to me for treatment of yellow lumps under his skin. They turned out to be cholesterol deposits, and they began to disappear a while after he started a low-fat diet I prescribed. He was so pleased with the results that he began to send his family and friends to me, and as a consequence I have watched over a small but loyal group of Chinese patients almost since the beginning of my practice. Unfortunately, many of them, especially the older ones, spoke only rudimentary English, a definite drawback for me in a field where obtaining a detailed history frequently leads directly to the diagnosis. The first several patients referred by Mr. Wong came to the office unaccompanied, usually holding a piece of paper with Chinese writing on it, probably my name and address. I had lots of time then, and it was a good thing, too, because it used to take me one or two hours just to find out what the patient's complaints were. Pantomime on both sides, together with the frequent use of the few English words that we had in common, finally more or less satisfied me, at least to the point where I could go on to the physical examination. Still, I must have missed many of the fine points that depend on sharing the same language, and since I was also not at all sure that they understood my recommendations, I began to feel more and more uncomfortable about the care that I was giving to these patients.

But then I had an idea. Maybe I could ask Mr. Wong to come to the office with those he recommended, at least those who were coming in for the first time, and to interpret for me. At first I was reluctant to ask, especially since I knew that he had to spend many hours a day in his one-man store, but he seemed pleased with my request and agreed without hesitation. We turned out to be a great team. He very quickly got the hang of the kind of detail I needed in both questions and answers, and after that my communication problems with Chinese patients were over.

He had open-heart surgery about fifteen years ago, but it was finally his worsening diabetes as well as the hardening of the arteries of his legs that pushed him into retirement from the import-export business. Yet even while he was still working, he never stopped coming in with every patient he recommended who might not be able to make himself understood. After his retirement, though, Mr. Wong expanded on this role and began to serve as the general liaison between "our" Chinese patients and me.

One day, he brought in Mr. Kiu, a restaurant owner from the neighborhood, for an initial visit. The patient had long-standing diabetes, and originally just wanted his blood sugar checked. With Mr. Wong's help, I was able to convince him that a complete checkup was in order. It was fortunate for him that he agreed, because not only did he turn out to have a large mass, which I found when I examined his rectum, but he also had an abnormal shadow on his chest x-ray. I explained to him that he had two problems that might or might not be related (his diabetes was apparently under control) and suggested a biopsy of the mass and a CAT scan of the chest, both of which could be done in the hospital before the one or two operations I thought he would need. Yet Mr. Kiu was due to go on vacation in several days and he refused to change his plans, despite eloquent pleas in Chinese and English by my liaison and me.

I was both furious and worried. But what made me even more furious than his stubbornness was that I was stuck with the worrying while he was, as far as I knew, enjoying himself. Three or four weeks went by. Mr. Wong contacted all his sources in the Chinese community but could not find out what had happened to our elusive patient. Meanwhile, fears of intestinal obstruction due to the rectal tumor (admittedly rare) or bleeding from the lung while Mr. Kiu was far from medical help frequently occupied my thoughts. And then he called one day. Acting as if we had been in agreement all along, he told me that he had had a wonderful vacation and that he was now ready to have "that rectal thing" taken care of. I explained that it was only prudent to investigate the lung shadow before going on to what was very likely going to be removal of part of his colon, but he refused. He went on to have surgery for his rectal cancer but never came back for follow-up after his discharge from the hospital. Even Mr. Wong, who rarely failed me in these matters, could not convince him to return. I had hoped to check his blood sugar again, and I had wanted to give the workup of the abnormal chest x-ray another try, but I finally had to admit that Mr. Kiu was a lost cause. My friend and adviser, Han Ming Wong, put it into perspective—but not, as one might expect, with a nugget of Oriental wisdom—when he said to me, "Forget him, Doc! You did your best, but what are you going to do? The guy's a jerk!"

Yet I cannot just shrug this kind of experience off. I would like to think (and, I admit, to make it appear to the world) that it is extreme conscientiousness that pushes me into trying to hold on to this kind of patient, despite his obviously impossible behavior. I am not alone in my persistence, though, since I have participated in some "can you top this?" contests in which my colleagues and I have competed for the title of who can stay the longest with the most difficult patient. It seems to me that we engage in these exercises in masochism because difficult patients test to the maximum the lessons that we have learned in medicine and that we would like to think make up our second skin: professionalism, compassion, and regard for the patient's feelings over our own. When I feel forced to finally give up, as I did with Mr. Kiu, I invariably feel empty and unfulfilled. It is possible that I turn the anger I feel toward the patient upon myself; after all, that is an accepted psychological mechanism. Still, under even these circumstances, I always think that I should have done better. With all my training—and, what's more, my extensive experience—why couldn't I prevail with a specific patient; for instance, Mr. Kiu? Could a more authoritative or a more diplomatic doctor have put his point across better? Maybe that doctor would not have ended up feeling that his patient had escaped from his care!

These are feelings, of course, and extreme ones at that. They usually have very little to do with the facts, but I describe them only because I want to demonstrate how at least one seemingly invincible man behind the desk can feel under these circumstances.

Fred Lane was a good old patient of mine who saw me about every two months after he had a ministroke several years before. His wife, Helen, a lady in her late fifties, was also my patient but never voiced a complaint either when she had one of her infrequent checkups or when she brought her husband to the office. But when she came to see me one day, telling me, "I feel terrible, and I'm never hungry anymore," I was immediately concerned. These vague symptoms are always disquieting for the doctor, especially if they are not accompanied by any other symptoms—in the abdomen or chest, for example, which would at least help to pinpoint the problem. What's more, since she had never been a "complainer," I had to take her statement at face value, and this made me even more alarmed. I was not surprised, however, when my checkup showed nothing wrong and that she had not even lost any weight. I had seen this kind of thing too often before: a serious illness that waits for a while to reveal itself. It had always seemed to me that the early warning system of the patient may not always hear the cries for help from his various organs before they do what they know best: enlarge or become smaller, grow bumps, and in the process agitate up to now tranquil laboratory tests and despoil previously virgin x-rays. I sensed very strongly that, sooner rather than later, we would see much more evidence of what was wrong. So I suggested that she take her temperature frequently, watch for any new symptoms, and keep in touch with me at least every other day. She seemed a little reassured by the good report, but still she looked worried, and I could not blame her. During the next several days, I thought about her case when I woke up in the middle of the night, as soon as I got up in the morning, and at odd times during the day. My top-priority obsessive thinking system had obviously been activated, an indication that my subconscious was also concerned about Mrs. Lane's diagnosis.

Three days later, she returned. Unfortunately, my subconscious and I had been correct. She now had shortness of breath, ankle swelling, and severe headaches that came and went. She agreed to be admitted to the diagnostic unit of the hospital, but this was the point where we had our first difficulty. Although her laboratory tests were again normal, she clearly had to have a nuclear magnetic resonance test (MRI) of her head as part of the workup for the cause of her headaches. She also needed a CAT scan of the abdomen because of her loss of appetite and ankle swelling.

It is well known that some patients can become claustrophobic during an MRI, since they are surrounded by a sort of cylinder during the procedure. Mrs. Lane could not tolerate the procedure from the very beginning but refused sedation, which usually relieves the anxiety symptoms, and for good measure adamantly rejected the CAT scan as well. Meanwhile, the hospital chest x-ray had shown an abnormality in the right lung. A CAT scan of the lung would, of course, have been very helpful in figuring out the cause of the abnormality. But she would not hear of it, so I was forced to suggest to her that we go directly to a bronchoscopy. I was surprised that she agreed to an invasive procedure when she had rejected several noninvasive ones, but as it happened, she tolerated the test very well. Nothing unusual was found on looking at the bronchi, and no abnormal cells were found in the biopsies or washings that were taken. I had in the meantime been able to convince her to undergo a sound wave test of the heart, and this showed nothing to suggest heart failure as the cause of the swelling and breathing problems. So there we were, still without a diagnosis; the patient's headaches were becoming more and more severe, and her ankles larger every time I looked at them.

Understandably, there were far fewer smiles from the Lanes for me than in the past, but I must admit that I also felt much less friendly toward them. I was very resentful because they had tied one diagnostic arm behind my back. What's more, I had suggested the next best thing to diagnosis, a trial of some medications to see if they would improve her symptoms, and they had refused those, too. I asked a neurologist and a lung specialist to see her, and both told me that they needed the procedures Mrs. Lane had refused in order to make a diagnosis. I felt absolutely boxed in. I had many talks with the patient and her family and I got nowhere with my suggestions. Finally, the patient asked me to discharge her: "I want to see how I get along at home." I was relieved in a sense because I would no longer have to face this frustrating situation every day. Yet her leaving did nothing to take away the anger and disappointment. If only she had allowed me to do what I knew how to do! Maybe then I could have clarified this puzzling clinical picture and, most important of all, relieved her suffering.

About a week later, I received a telephone call from an internist on the staff of another prestigious Manhattan medical center. He was seeing Mrs. Lane and could not see why she had had a bronchoscopy without a prior CAT scan, why she had had no study of her head, and so on and so on. He sounded somewhat indignant, but I could tell that he was also just the slightest bit pleased that someone in a hospital that in recent years had begun to outshine his own had done such an evidently poor job. As everybody, and not just patients, will often do, Mrs. Lane must have told him her story without mentioning her own negative role in the whole affair. I told the doctor what I knew, but could not resist suggesting that he retake her history, this time with special emphasis on asking the patient the very questions that he had originally asked me.

Doctors do know better almost always. This is an undeniable void between patients and doctors that no amount of hostility, arrogance, or obstructive behavior can ever fill in. It should come as no great surprise, though, because, after all, we learn and practice and some of us teach medicine from our twenties on, to the exclusion of any other work. Decisions in medicine sometimes appear deceptively simple, so that patients may honestly believe that their own common sense or their expertise in their work entitles them to an equal voice in a medical dialogue with the doctor. This misunderstanding exists because patients truly do not know how we think and are not aware (perfectly justifiably) of the complicated considerations that go into decisions on *all* cases, no matter how elementary they appear at first glance.

Let's say, for instance, that a healthy middle-aged man has a fever for two days. On examination, he does not look particularly sick, and he has no cough, abdominal pain, or difficulties with urination, or any other symptoms that could give a hint about the source of the fever. As a matter of fact, the only thing that is sure about the whole case so far is that he wants to return to work as soon as possible. What is more reasonable to the patient or his family than for him to be started on antibiotics? Yet my considerations are entirely different. I think that he very likely has a virus, in which case antibiotics would not help anyway. Yet I am not sufficiently sure of this diagnosis that I do not want to observe the temperature for another day or two. If it continues beyond that time, it is probably not caused by a garden-variety virus and the patient will require cultures, a chest x-ray, and so on. At *that* point, if a bacterial infection is shown to be at the bottom of the fever, a specific antibiotic can be given. What's more, a random antibiotic given earlier might have delayed the diagnosis by just taking the edge off the infection and giving falsely negative cultures.

I tell this story just to give a little insight into some of the factors that go into our decision making. Even the most sophisticated patient cannot be expected to have the kind of knowledge and judgment that most doctors possess. Since we are not only fallible but also human, even the best of us make mistakes, which we try from that moment on never to make again. And yes, there are some doctors who should not be practicing because they are incompetent, so that I wholeheartedly agree with a program of periodic retesting. Sooner or later, though, a patient will have to put himself in *some* physician's hands. It is at this point that he can best help himself by being a cooperative and intelligent participant in his own care, while allowing the professionally trained and experienced pilot to fly the airplane.

There are many occasions, though, when patients just plain resist giving up their autonomy. Strangely enough, many of these patients readily go along with the doctor's advice but are unwilling to accept what they perceive as his dominant role in the relationship. So they snipe away at the doctor about matters that have nothing to do with medicine but everything to do with temperament. They criticize the decor of his office, the manners of his staff, even the color combination that he wears on a particular day. It always comes down to the same issue, though: these people cannot tolerate *being* patients, something that can only mean to them dependency and loss of control.

Sarah Dillman was my patient for about the last ten years I

was in practice. She came in regularly for checkups and never rejected any of my recommendations. Yet every time she came to see me, she spent at least half the office visit on a detailed description of what she did not like about my office. Although her manner was otherwise charming, there was an insistent and aggressive note to her criticism that irritated me from the very beginning. I freely admit that the place where I saw my patients was not at all elegant, and it is true that it could have used a painting and some new carpets. But it was clean and quite efficient, although it looked chaotic, since files and equipment were wedged into every available little space. I have always been against especially fancy doctors' offices. While I am sure that patients are impressed by leather, fine wood, and chrome, it should be apparent to them that their fees pay for this elaborate show rather than, let us say, for more advanced diagnostic equipment. Come to think of it, I never provided piped-in music or television in my waiting room, either, because I have always believed that the place where serious matters of health and life are discussed should have a dignified atmosphere and should not be mistaken for an airport lounge or an elevator.

But Sarah never let up in her attacks, using terms like *chintzy*, *dismal*, and even *slum*. I had heard from others that she had exquisite taste and lived in a beautifully furnished apartment, but I realized very early on that it was not my office decor that was the problem. I felt, rather, that before obeying my medical suggestions, she had the need to cut me down to size, and that insulting the place where I worked was as good a way as any to achieve that. One day, as she was launching into her usual tirade, I could not help but show my anger. I know that I should have tried to give her insight into her motives instead, but I did not think that she was psychologically equipped for this kind of explanation. Besides, her repeated criticism, which really had a malicious edge to it, had gotten under my skin. I gave her a choice: either she stopped her complaints about my office or she got herself another doctor. From then on, she left her design objections at home and never brought the subject up again. Obviously, I do not look back on this event as a victory, and I am still a little ashamed that I lost my temper. Maybe she was testing me all the while and got whatever emotional satisfaction she needed by *making* me put my foot down, just that once.

What the doctor calls the patient, and vice versa, also has to do with power. Calling some patients by their first names has been with us for generations and was not considered unusual until recently. Of course, the practice has always been discriminatory. Women, minorities, and patients in municipal hospitals were always more likely to be treated in this patronizing manner, while corporation CEOs or lawyers, for example, rarely suffered this indignity. I am as guilty of this as anyone in my generation, and when I think back on it, I find it difficult to understand why the unfairness of it did not strike me much earlier. Young doctors nowadays are more respectful of *all* patients, and we, the older ones, have learned from them. More than occasionally, though, a patient will ask the doctor to call him by his first name. It may make him feel more secure or more protected, so I see nothing wrong in going along with his wish.

What to call someone in today's world is assuming less and less importance. Yet how a patient addresses his doctor has a significance all its own and has nothing to do with empty formalities or with etiquette. Ideally, the relationship between a doctor and his patient should have a certain amount of distance built into it, which then separates it from the uncertain attitudes of acquaintanceship or friendship. The patient who, right from the beginning, calls the doctor by his first name, though, is trying to get around this natural obstacle. In his own mind, he is transforming the doctor into a friend and in this way knocks out any obligation to "obey" him. Yet at least some degree of authority is absolutely necessary if the doctor is to be effective in his role. If the patient, even if he does it unconsciously, reduces him to the status of a well-informed friend, he does himself a disservice.

How do you handle this touchy situation? I have found that the least embarrassing way is not to draw attention to what the patient is doing but just to continue calling him by his last name and not be drawn into the invitation "Call me by my first name, too." Going into explanations about what he is really trying to do is really useless and just serves to make the patient resentful. He usually gets the hint rather quickly, though, and most often does not realize that what appears to him to be just stiffness and excessive formality on the doctor's part was really instrumental in putting the relationship back on the right track.

I had my most bizarre experience in the never-ending struggle we have with our patients for power and control about ten years ago with a new patient, a woman in her early forties. Although many other doctors do it differently, it was my custom to first see a new patient in the examining room, after blood had already been drawn and an electrocardiogram and chest x-ray had been done. The patient, by this point, would already be undressed and wearing an examining gown. After I had taken the history and performed the physical examination, I would ask the patient to get dressed and we would then talk about my findings while sitting across from each other in my consultation room. Very occasionally, a patient objected to having any procedures done before meeting me, and after I had introduced myself and explained the office routine, the problem was almost always resolved. My secretary, Marian, had an uncanny instinct for picking up hostility or strange behavior in patients from the time they first called up to their actual arrival in the office. In these situations, she usually gave me plenty of warning, so that by the time I saw the patient I was well prepared for all eventualities. In this case, though, no news from Marian was good news, and I entered the examining room without any preconceived notions.

I always have a little bit of stage fright when I see a new patient. It is not that I do not welcome the challenge, because I really do. Besides, I have never seen a patient for the first time where I did not anticipate the possibility of seeing something I had never seen before or of making a great diagnosis of which I had only dreamed in the past. What frightens me is purely a matter of vanity. Will the patient I am going to see be disappointed, or will she agree with the high grades given to me by the friend who referred her? Or: I have been a little down recently. Will the patient pick it up and be discouraged about sticking with me? The comparison with acting is apt, because just as an actor can be perfectly competent and still flop, a doctor can do and think all the right things and still not "come across." It seems to me that what I am really talking about is what used to be called bedside manner. Looking back on the number of patients I saw in my medical lifetime and the feedback I got from them, I am quite sure that I had it. But just as the doctor is constantly evaluating the patient, emotionally as well as physically, so the patient checks the doctor for alertness, interest, consistency in his opinions, and so on. After a while, we build up credit with our established patients, and they give us a little bit of leeway on the occasions when we are not at our best. But a new patient has no means of comparison, and often we have only one shot at them before they make up their minds about us. But then again, is it not normal for some patients to just not like us on first sight? Of course it is, and it happens in the outside world all the time. It is just a measure of our insecurity, and therefore of my stage fright, that what we really yearn for (but deep down know we cannot have) is 100 percent acceptance by *all* our patients, past, present, and future.

The patient looked ill at ease sitting on the examining table. The room was warm, but she had her coat on over her paper gown, and although she volunteered her name, Barbara Mautner, she did not wait for me to introduce myself before she began to speak. Her voice was tight, as if she were barely able to control herself. I noticed immediately that her hands were shaking, and I wondered whether this was due to an overactive thyroid or, given her obvious agitation, whether it did not just come from excitement. I quickly decided on the latter possibility.

She furiously complained of "being treated like a piece of meat," of being "thrown" into an examining room and "ordered" to undress without any regard whatsoever for her feelings. I was happy to see that her electrocardiogram was on the little desk and that her chest x-ray had already been developed and was mounted on the illuminated view box. Patients always appreciated my prompt attention to these worrisome items and they were usually much more relaxed if they knew, right from the beginning, that they were not matters for concern. I looked at the films carefully and read the tracing, and I interrupted her with the good news that I saw nothing wrong with either one. I added, before she could resume her speech, that one of the reasons for my seeing the patient after the procedures had been done was my desire to take the tension out of the waiting for results.

My reassurances did nothing to pacify her, however, and she finally came to what was really bothering her—that she had had to get undressed. I then asked her how she had resolved this problem with her other physicals, and it turned out that she had never had one during her entire adult life. She then asked me what I was going to do, and I explained my usual procedure. "Why do I have to be totally undressed?" she asked, and I replied that a thorough examination required access to the *whole* body and not just small areas that the patient chose to reveal.

So far, the conversation was not outside my experience. Some patients—mostly women, but occasionally men as well—are unusually reluctant to expose any part of their bodies for scrutiny. This is widely interpreted as shyness or self-consciousness but is mostly not confined to strictly medical situations. These people do not like to be seen in the nude by spouses or lovers, either, and the reasons for this fear are not relevant here. Yet the inhibitions of these patients have never forced me to hold off from examining them. As a matter of fact, this kind of situation stimulated me to be much more patient than I usually was (not very, I confess freely) and to "talk the patient through" each step by describing what I was going to do and the reason for doing it. In this way, I made the patient a much more active participant in the examination. Of course, I did not expect a basic change in attitude just because of this one experience, but at least I was able to do what I had to do, and the patient's cooperation, though hesitant at first, made all the difference.

Mrs. (wedding ring evident) Mautner was not interested in being helped in the way I just described. It was at this point that I realized something else was going on and that I might be going into uncharted territory. But her next statement, although startling, made everything very clear, and I realized that her maneuver was just a variation on the familiar power game. What she said was this: "Either I get dressed right now and only uncover the part of me I'll *let* you examine, or you get undressed also, and that will make us equal." What she said makes her sound a little crazy, but I think it was just an extreme way of showing that she was not going to give up control. We had reached an impasse. Going along with her first condition would have seriously compromised the examination, and the second one was there just for provocation's sake. Judging from our initial meeting, there was no way I could take care of this lady in a reasonable fashion. I suggested that she do what she so fervently wished to do (that is, get dressed) and find herself another doctor.

The question of who is in charge, the doctor or the patient, is not likely to ever go away. We doctors feel very strongly that, in order to be able to do our very best for our patients, they must in turn let us do what we have to do with a minimum of interference. On the other hand, we patients cannot bear to give a blank check to just anyone, no matter how many certificates he has on his wall, when the issue is our life.

Doctors and their patients cannot do without each other, that's for sure. "Managing illness" is an impersonal term that does not begin to describe our delicate interaction. The ill totally depend upon doctors for reassurance, relief of pain, an understanding of what is wrong with them, and, they hope, effective treatment. Yet without patients our mission does not exist, our training is wasted, and our experience counts for nothing. We recognize that we have to live with each other, but how agreeably we do that depends upon the circumstances. Sometimes it is the doctor who is obviously "winning" and can therefore afford to act fatherly and be magnanimous. At other times, it is the patient who has prevailed. He has successfully avoided "obeying" but he has not burned his bridges with the doctor, because he has at least appeared cooperative. This is politics at its most intricate, and it would be fascinating in its own right if the stakes were not so high. I do not believe that whether medical decisions (all crucial, by the way, whether they apply to a cold or to a cancer) are implemented or not should have to depend on such vague notions as the forceful personality, or the tendency to "bossiness," or the "difficult nature," or, for that matter, the innate passivity of the patient or doctor. There is no substitute for straight talk between both sides in order to resolve this eternal conflict. This is often difficult to achieve, though, because doctors can be touchy and patients tend to be intimidated by such discussions. Yet I do not know what else to suggest. If we are ever to get beyond the chaotic system of decision making that is the only one we know, many patients are going to have to open up and be more forthright about what is bothering them, and not leave one doctor after another just to avoid unpleasant dialogues. And doctors are going to have to learn what is so foreign to many of them, that if they expect their patients to respect their decisions and recommendations, they will have to explain and convince rather than forcibly impose their views.

3

Money

DURING THE FIRST YEAR I was in practice, a lady in her early seventies by the name of Pearl Berkowitz became my patient. I do not remember if she was referred by a friend or by another doctor, what her problem was, or what she looked like, but I have thought of her often in the last thirty years. She had been under my care for several months when *she called and asked to see me as soon as possible "for a talk."* I knew that she lived in Coney Island, at the far end of Brooklyn, and that it would take one or two hours for her to get to my office in the East Thirties in Manhattan. Obviously, she had something important to talk about, and I told my secretary to tell her to come right over, however long it took to get there. I wondered what it was that she thought was so important that it could not be discussed over the telephone and so urgent that she was willing to brave the subway during rush hour. Had I antagonized her in some way, and did she mean to go to another physician? I doubted it, not only because she had always praised me for being thorough and for giving her a lot of my time, but also because patients almost never *personally* inform the doctor that they are quitting his care. They find it difficult and embarrassing even under harmonious circumstances to have an in-depth talk with "their" doctor, let alone when they are so unhappy with him that they want to switch to someone else. Because of this, they find it easier instead to drop out of sight without a word, or to send a release for the transfer of their records without an added explanation.

Or did she have something that alarmed her so much that she needed to describe it at length before allowing me to examine the breast lump or the mole she had found? Maybe; I had seen this before with patients who instinctively know they have something worrisome and will do anything to delay the fearsome diagnosis for even a brief time.

Of course, I did not spend the next hours concentrating solely on the possible reasons for Mrs. Berkowitz's impending visit, but I describe my thoughts in order to give some insight into the obsessive notions that we doctors are prone to. Because we have seen the worst so often, we have to keep it within our reach, we cannot deny it, it is part of our inventory. Yet even just the suggestion of the abyss sends us scurrying back to safer ground and makes us wish for a happy outcome. Are we, then, to be called fearful optimists or hopeful pessimists? I think we are the latter.

When she finally sat across from me at my desk late in the day, it became obvious, very quickly, that she was neither sick nor harboring anything against me personally. She then hesitated for a long time before she admitted that "money trouble" was the reason for her visit and that she had wanted to see me as soon as possible because she was so upset. This confession surprised me since she had never questioned my fees, nor had she ever failed to pay in full at the time of her visits. But I knew that she was a retired garment worker and that she had a modest Blue Shield plan (this was in the days before Medicare). Before she even got around to the exact nature of her financial problem, I offered to reduce the fees (which were not all that high to begin with) my office would charge her in the future. She thanked me for my kindness but refused. She then said something that made such an impression on me that I remember it word for word: "Doctor, you are a very good doctor, but in the long run I won't be able to afford you! Could you maybe refer me to a *less* good doctor?"

I knew that I needed time to reflect on her startling question, but in the meantime I again offered to change my fees for her. She was adamant in her refusal, saying: "Doctor, I didn't come all this way to bargain with you. I came to tell you how much I think of what you do and that you deserve to get the money that you charge. For me to pay you less would mean that you are *worth* less, so I can't do that!"

When we parted, she kissed my hand. She belonged to the generation of Eastern Europeans who still did that when they wanted to show affection and respect for the doctor, and I was very moved by the gesture. I referred her to a friend of mine who had also trained at Bellevue and who was practicing in Brooklyn. Yet I had not gone along completely with her request. Although his fees were lower, he was not a less good doctor than I.

Of course, Pearl Berkowitz was a product of her immigrant upbringing. She had learned that quality costs, but also that you do not undertake obligations you cannot afford. So she looked at my care as she would at a new winter coat or a lamp for her living room and made a conscious decision to go for something cheaper, although she obviously regretted having to make the choice. When I realized that I could not make her change her mind, I tried my best to make things as easy as possible for her. I knew that she must have been very embarrassed by the whole episode, especially because patients in those days were even more reluctant than now to expose their feelings to their doctors.

Nowadays, paying for medical care has become a matter for politicians, economists, and those scavengers, the insurance companies. Individual patients watch while the titans confer, and they can only hope that all this benevolent attention does not, as is sometimes seen in medicine, make the cure worse than the disease.

Nobody likes to spend money, and especially when it is for services and not for something tangible like a good steak, a car, or a television set. Yet people especially resent having to pay for medical care. This resentment is felt by the poor *and* the rich, the stingy as well as the generous, and in my experience has even come up when the patient has had no out-of-pocket expense at all and the entire bill has been paid by the insurance company.

Yet I think the issue of *having* to pay a doctor for his services goes way beyond the actual exchange of money. I have always felt that patients view the caring, the reassurance, and the sympathy they expect from us to be the equivalent of the nurturing they got (or at least hoped to get) as children from their parents. Later in life, when they find that they have to pay for the feeling of being protected, for the luxury of having someone who cares make hard decisions for them, for turning on the light when the darkness of anxiety is all around, it is a bitter pill for them to swallow.

There is also another reason for the resentment so many patients and their families feel against doctors. Probably because of the peculiar aspects of what we do and the very intimate nature of the relationship we have with our patients, I have found that they are fascinated with where we live, what kind of car we drive, what our wives look like, and so on. The "Dr." in front of the name, the M.D. plates on the car, and being paged in public places all make us much more highly visible than, let us say, an insurance company executive or a lawyer. This unavoidable loss of at least part of our anonymity makes it much easier for the public to satisfy its curiosity about us and to dislike us for what looks like a "highfalutin" way of life.

Some years ago, the *New York Times* was doing an article about unusual New York apartments and asked my wife and me if it could include ours. We had spent an enormous amount of effort, not to speak of a great deal of money, on the renovation of what had been a "wreck," and we were proud of what we had accomplished. We saw no reason not to agree, so several weeks later the article appeared. It was short, several other apartments were discussed as well, and it ran on one of the back pages on a weekday. Our name was mentioned, but the fact that I am a doctor was omitted. In the next weeks, it seemed to me that everyone I knew or had ever known had seen the article and mentioned it to me. Acquaintances and colleagues at the hospital were generally positive, or at least appeared to be. What was so revealing, though, was the response of my patients. My wife and I had begun to have some qualms about what they would say after we already had given permission to the newspaper to use our apartment for the article. Yet I was not prepared for the extent and the unanimity of the response. With very few exceptions, every patient who spoke to me about the article, and there were some who wrote as well, had something to say that mixed admiration with a darker sentiment. "I guess the heart attack I had two years ago really helped to make that apartment so beautiful!" was a typical response. Another not infrequent comment was, I guess, supposed to warn me about the future: "I hope you don't fix up another apartment soon; your fees are high enough as it is!"

I should really have known better than to go public, however innocently, with something having to do with my personal life. I was hurt by these statements, but I was not really surprised. I have known for a very long time that, emotionally, patients cannot separate the money they pay the doctor for services rendered from the reason that made the services necessary in the first place. It looks to them as if their illness financed a specific, small piece of the doctor's economic well-being, and that their suffering served, let us say, to buy the leather upholstery for the doctor's Mercedes or an antique chair for his apartment. None of my patients was completely negative (at least to my face) when commenting about the article. Their rational selves understood—reluctantly, I am sure—that their doctor has the same right as they do to live as he chooses. Yet this response to the publicity about my apartment also made me understand something I had not thought about before. Patients also feel exploited, on a deeper level, because they have the impression that it is in the doctor's best interests for his patients to be sick; otherwise he might not live nearly as well as he does.

Of course, this is an emotional response, and it is even understandable. The reality, though, is that disease is unfortunately so much a part of our existence that we do not have to resort to wishing it on our patients. Not that we would anyway, but I find it very hard to imagine the average doctor coming into his office in the morning, reviewing the bills he has to pay, and saying to himself: "Boy, I hope twenty of my patients get sick today and come to see me. I can't hold off paying the mortgage any longer!" On the other hand, there is nothing wrong with hoping to be called for a consultation or two in the hospital, or by a patient for his annual checkup, on a day when the appointment book is discouragingly meager. Except for doctors who are psychopaths and criminals (and who should energetically be weeded out of our profession), I think it is safe to say that the rest of us would never wish harm on a patient *whatever* the motive.

Appropriately enough, doctors are conflicted as well, and have difficulty in justifying the charging of fees, especially early in the game. They are on salary during their training period and thus have no financial relationship with their patients. When he leaves his residency, the fledgling practitioner is insecure about charging for what he has always done for free, so that the transition from trainee to reluctant businessman is a shocking one. Worse yet, he is puzzled by how he can justify charging for being compassionate and caring and for using the expertise taught, not sold, him at the bedside of sick people. And what's more, doesn't the whole concept get reduced to the absurd if we try to put a certain dollar value on, say, one day's worth of continuous concern felt by a conscientious doctor about his very sick patient?

There is no escaping the fact that money is an unfortunate side issue in the already very tense relationship between patients and doctors. Yet just attacking surface issues having to do with obvious money matters will not solve the deeper problems, which are based on fantasy and misconceptions. The patient is in a bind. He has conflicted emotions about paying for love, but his sense of reality tells him that if he is ever to get medical care, he will have to pay the price of admission. The doctor, on the other hand, would ideally like to concentrate fully on taking care of his patients and not be distracted by the constraints of running a small business; yet he wants to make a good living as well. Nevertheless, he has to come to grips with the fact that, even if he works for a group, an HMO, or a hospital (which just makes him part of a bigger business), the patient somehow has to be charged for his services. How else can he practice good medicine, which requires such essentials as a clean and decently appointed office, and proper help and diagnostic equipment? And how is his way of life going to be financed? After many years of study and financial sacrifice, a comfortable middle-class to upper-middle-class way of life is not an unrealistic goal for a young doctor. What's more, it is to the patient's advantage if his doctor does not feel forced to cut corners or to see an excessive number of patients because of economic need.

In banking and in business, for example, money is what it's all about. However, when we talk about medicine or any other service where money does not buy something that can be wrapped up and taken home, or driven, or lived in, it can easily create controversy. Then the whole problem comes down to the *perception* of the service by either party. Patients, like all consumers, do not want to be made to look like fools. They have legitimate concerns, such as, for instance, the amount of time the doctor spends with them, whether the fees they are being charged are reasonable, whether they are being billed for a service that was not actually performed, and so on.

Before even going into these issues, though, I have to admit something that is, of course, very well known but that is a very painful issue for many physicians. There are some real thieves in the doctor population! They charge outrageous fees, cheat insurance companies, sell prescriptions for drugs, and do not give quality care although they charge for it, also a form of thievery. The possession of an M.D. degree in no way guarantees an exemption from criminal tendencies or behavior, and the patients, as usual, are the ultimate victims of these unscrupulous doctors.

Yet my experience tells me that many of the objections that patients raise about paying for medical care have nothing to do with shady practices on the part of the doctor. The same goes for any number of just plain mistakes made in billing either by hand or by computer, which have made me offer my share of embarrassed apologies to patients over the years. But still, crooked doctors and inadvertent errors cause just a small percentage of the complaints made by patients when they receive that little time bomb, the doctor's bill, in the mail.

The patient, understandably, wants to know whether a particular service (for instance, a prolonged office visit, a visit in the intensive care unit, or a consultation in the emergency room at two A.M.) is "worth" the fee that he is charged. Yet most of the time there is no reasonable answer to this question, not only because of our peculiar billing system but also because patients do not ever know what we really do and how long it takes for us to do it. Lawyers charge by the hour, so that the more complicated the case, the more time is billed to the client. The hourly fee is discussed in advance, and although "sticker shock" does occur, it is usually confined to surprise at the number of hours billed rather than the hourly fee itself.

In contrast, we doctors charge by the visit or by the operation. A surgeon will bill the same amount for a particular operation—let us say, a coronary bypass—whether it takes him four hours or eight hours, and whether, in the postoperative period, the patient requires many visits or his convalescence is completely uncomplicated. I admit that psychiatrists mostly charge by the hour (really fifty minutes, the only human influence on time that I have ever heard of), but the fees charged by the rest of us are figured in a very haphazard way and have very little to do with the time actually spent.

Aside from tradition ("We've always done it this way" must have been the catchphrase in medicine since the beginning), we are reluctant to charge strictly for our time because that would often frighten our patients. I realize that it sounds far-fetched, but try to imagine the following: Early in the evening, before going home, I visit a sixty-four-year-old lady who is in the hospital for an angiogram. She has recently had chest pain more frequently than before, although it is always quickly relieved by nitroglycerin taken under the tongue. Earlier in the afternoon, the usual pain was not relieved by *several* nitroglycerins, although it ultimately disappeared on its own. My physical examination shows nothing new. The EKG technician is busy elsewhere, and I cannot find the intern. It takes me ten minutes to find a machine, and then I do the electrocardiogram myself. It shows no change from those done recently, yet I am suspicious that the patient may be starting to close off one of her coronary arteries. I want to transfer her to the coronary care unit, but this cannot be done without a discussion with the resident. It takes fifteen minutes for him to call me back after I page him, and when he does, he tells me that since there is no vacant bed in the unit, my patient's transfer will have to wait until someone else can be moved out. While I am trying to make arrangements, I look in on the patient a few times and am glad that she looks stable and that she has had no further pain. I also call her husband to inform him of what is going on. I then call the consulting cardiologist, who cannot immediately be located. While I am waiting for the intern and resident to come (although she appears all right, she needs direct supervision by a doctor on the floor until she is transferred to the coronary care unit), I realize that the cardiologist has not called back yet. When the resident arrives and I again find that she is stable, I feel that it is safe for me to go home, which is nearby. As soon as I arrive, the cardiologist is on the phone and I discuss the situation with him for a few minutes. During the evening, I speak to the resident three times about the patient's general condition and the results of the preliminary blood tests. By this time, her electrocardiogram shows evidence of a heart attack.

At three A.M., the intern calls to tell me that the monitor shows many extra beats and that her blood pressure has dropped slightly. We agree on a medication to use against the extra beats and decide to just watch the blood pressure. I wake up at six A.M., earlier than usual, probably because my patient has been on my mind all night, and I know then that my anxiety will be relieved only if I go to see her now, which I do.

If I billed the patient for the time I actually spent, she would probably not only be surprised but worried as well. I might easily not have spent more than fifteen minutes physically with her during this entire time, yet I probably occupied myself with her situation for another several hours. A charge for the total time spent would not only be much higher than the standard hospital visit fee, it might also make the patient question my honesty, since the time she actually saw me was so limited. The most important thing, though, is that an exact breakdown of the time I spent on her case would very likely have made the patient quite anxious. Even looking back, I feel it was really not necessary for her to realize by reading her bill how much care she needed—in other words, how sick she had really been.

It seems more than a coincidence that quite a few patients used to complain about receiving a bill from one or another of the doctors who covered for me during my free time by saying, "He just stood at the door for a couple of minutes, asked me how I was, and left. Then I got a bill for . . ." I would look at the notes in the chart and usually found that these doctors had included some fact that could have been obtained only through physical examination, which meant that the doctor could not just have waved from the door. Was I supposed to believe that *all* my covering doctors wrote dishonest reports? Hardly, although it is certainly possible that an occasional one cut some corners on a busy weekend. Were the patients all liars? Of course not, but I believe that the resentment about money matters that is just under the surface with all patients often has a way of distorting the facts, so that supposed exploitation by doctors becomes a self-fulfilling prophecy.

But what if you are seen by a doctor just for a cold, let us say, and he spends only five minutes with you? He looks as if he knows what he is doing, he checks your temperature himself, he examines your throat and ears, he has you take your shirt or blouse off so that he can listen to your chest. He then gives you a prescription and asks you to call by the next day if you are not better. His charge seems high. So many dollars for five min- utes! But don't forget that there is no extra fee if you call him tonight because you cannot breathe, or if you have to speak to him tomorrow because your temperature is not down. Yet even if you get better quickly, and he really had to spend only five minutes with you, it is very probable that, at another time, the same fee will cover a more complicated situation. In other words, when it comes to doctors' services, time and money usually average out over the long run.

The public is justly suspicious of doctors "covering up" for each other. With our specialized knowledge and our close emo- tional ties to our colleagues, we are certainly capable of pulling the wool over our patients' eyes. I could be called naive and blind to much more widespread dishonesty on the part of doc- tors, but I sincerely believe that this is not the case. As I have said before, there are crooked doctors, and they rob the patients by charging them (and their insurance companies) while not giving value in return. I admit also that doctors are not only poor businessmen but tend to be gullible as well. This is how they often open themselves up to charges of greed and ethically marginal practices. But don't forget that the public feels a certain satisfaction in witnessing the tearing down, at least a little bit, of the reputation of their doctors, a group that used to be considered very special and, in certain ways, untouchable. The newspapers know very well how to present the fall from grace of a doctor in the most dramatic fashion. It is fully understandable, then, how an already resentful public, with financial problems of its own, is willing to assume the worst about our whole profession based on what are usually very isolated cases.

There are wide swings in the "worth" that the patient and his family attach to a doctor's services. Before the diagnosis is made, which I have found to be the time when the patient experiences the greatest anxiety, "I'll pay *anything* if I'm okay" is a refrain we hear frequently. After the operation, or after the tests are back and the patient knows what he has, no matter whether the news is good or bad, this *"anything"* has a way of being drastically reduced downward.

My father, who has been a doctor for sixty-five of his ninety-one years (I have been a doctor for only thirty-six years), sums up his own experience with these predictable ups and downs by saying, "There is a very good reason why prostitutes ask for their money in advance. Afterward, when everything that was supposed to happen happened, the value of the transaction to the client just isn't the same anymore!"

He told me a story years ago that illustrates this point but applies more to our profession than to the one he referred to in his little saying. One of his professors, Heinrich von Neumann, was the best-known ear, nose, and throat specialist in Vienna during the 1920s. One night, he was urgently called to the home of the Argentinian ambassador, whose child had swallowed a fish bone. He rushed over in his fiacre—his horse-drawn carriage—and was ushered into the dining room of the embassy, which was in a complete uproar. A lady who was evidently the child's mother was sitting in a corner and shrieking in Spanish; the servants were running back and forth, calling to each other in their Viennese dialect; and two other children were sitting on the floor, ignored and crying. The patient, a six-year-old boy, was breathing in noisy little gasps and already had blue lips, a sign of oxygen lack. He was limp in the arms of his father, who was pacing back and forth and occasionally slapping him on the back (an abortive Heimlich maneuver so long ago?). Von Neumann knew that the child was about to die, and so, without any preliminary examination whatsoever, he pried the boy's mouth open and stuck his legendarily long right index finger (his left one was evidently of normal size) into the little boy's throat. Everyone became very still as he performed a little rotating maneuver with his finger and then jerked it back. A gleaming white needlelike object, the offending fish bone, came out of the child's mouth as if glued to the end of the doctor's forefinger. At this moment, the room became even noisier than before as the patient, his lips and his face pinking up noticeably, began to cry. His mother had resumed her shrieking, but now with joy, and his father kept walking the child around the room as if in a daze. Von Neumann, having been called away just as he was about to drink his after-dinner demitasse, sat down at the table and asked one of the servants to bring him a cup of black coffee. After a few minutes, the ambassador was composed enough to sit down with him to discuss the fee. Pulling fish bones out of dying little children was evidently not the professor's only talent, because he then said something unforgettable that is just as valid now as it was then: "Why don't you just pay me *half* of what you were going to pay me if I pulled out the fish bone, but when it was still in your little boy's throat!"

Of course, we appreciate patients who do not argue about their bills and pay promptly. What they are saying with their cooperative behavior is that they feel we are doing a good job and that it is only right to pay us for it. Like any other business (I always use this word reluctantly when it applies to medicine, but I must), a medical practice needs cash flow to survive. The rent must be paid, employees must get their salaries on time, and the doctor himself must pay for personal expenses, just to name several of the larger items in the weekly check-writing ceremony, which is the very opposite of TGIF. Happily, almost every practice has its share of the "good" patients, the ones who pay with a minimum of fuss, and they are the financial backbone for what is usually an otherwise not very sound economic entity. This does not at all mean that the patients who are conscientious about paying are in any way "patsies." These people are usually very alert and are not afraid to question anything that does not appear correct; what they do not do, though, is use money as a weapon against the doctor.

Surprisingly, the outright "bad" patients, the ones who run out on the bill, are not a major problem. They usually steal (isn't it stealing when you decide, usually in advance, not to pay for something that is done for you?) one office visit or checkup from you, and then they never come back. No matter how computerized it is and how efficiently it is run, no practice has a 100 percent collection rate; nor do we expect one. Doctors can accept, philosophically, an occasional robbery of their services. Yet they are terribly frustrated by the patient who keeps coming around, all the while arguing about his bill and at the same time minimizing the quality of what was done for him. This attempt to lower the value of the service, *which has already been rendered*, is almost always a trick designed to save money, but it makes doctors terribly resentful. They look at this maneuver as something that shows a lack of appreciation for what they have done, and in their eyes that is a much more serious issue than the financial one could ever be. Most doctors I know, including myself, do not hesitate to lower fees or to cancel them altogether if they feel the patient has a genuine problem in paying. But when I have done my work conscientiously and encounter the sort of behavior that might be acceptable at a flea market or wherever else bargaining and downgrading of the product is a fact of life, I do not give in. This may appear hard-hearted and unnecessarily rigid, but as I have said, at this point it is no longer about money; it *is* about the work that I have done, and I refuse to minimize the value of that.

*   *   *

There is another type of patient, however, who makes the ones I have described so far seem cooperative in comparison. Mr. Sherman was a man in his fifties who came to see me because of increasing weakness. He was in the fur business and claimed that he had been referred by a client of his, whose name he had forgotten. Right off the bat he told me how much he appreciated now being under my care (he had investigated me, he said, and had heard very positive things about me) and also that he had wanted someone on the staff of my particular hospital, "where there are so many good doctors." He turned out to be anemic, with very poor kidney function, and I suggested that he be hospitalized for further investigation and, probably, a kidney biopsy. He agreed, and since hospital care nowadays, as we all know, can be shockingly expensive, I asked him whether he was covered by insurance. He laughed and said, "All kinds!" He added, "Doctor, I can afford it. I want the very best! Call all the specialists you want; *money is no object!*" This last statement gave me a vague feeling of discomfort. I had heard it quite a few times before, and I had found on each occasion that money was no object because the patient was not intending to pay in the first place. I had no choice, though. No matter what my suspicions were, he was sick and required care, and he was now my responsibility.

Mr. Sherman was hospitalized for the next seven weeks. He had a kidney biopsy, and ultimately he needed frequent dialysis for what turned out to be a chronic nephritis, or kidney inflammation. I felt that consultations with a nephrologist, a urologist, and a hematologist were in order and that our dialysis expert should see him on a regular basis. However, the patient requested many more consultations on his own for complaints I easily could have handled myself. He asked me to call a gastroenterologist because he had heartburn (a common symptom in kidney failure, by the way), a lung specialist because he had an occasional cough, a dermatologist because of a minor rash on his back, and so on. After a few weeks, my secretary began to receive calls from some of the consultants' secretaries, who had received no checks in response to the bills they had sent to him. Speaking to a patient or a family about money during an illness that still requires hospitalization is a very sensitive subject. In Mr. Sherman's case, it was doubly difficult because he was single, so that there was not even any family to contact. Even if the doctor is convinced that it is perfectly safe, at a certain moment, to discuss the payment of medical bills, he opens himself up to accusations of "harassment," "insensitivity," and "money grubbing," to name just a few of the charges I have heard leveled at other doctors as well as myself over the years. Yet, as I have said before, time has a way of diminishing the patient's enthusiasm for the doctor's services. So it makes sense to at least discuss payment while still seeing the patient every day, before he goes home and the whole episode, including, understandably, what the doctor has done, recedes into that remote niche in memory that is reserved for particularly unpleasant experiences.

Mr. Sherman was perfectly pleasant when I took the right opportunity to speak to him about the other doctors' bills. I had decided not to speak to him about my own yet (I had seen him once or twice a day for six weeks by then) because I was waiting to see how he would react to the payment of *any* bills. "Doctor," he said, "my finances are all screwed up. I don't even know what my bank balance is! The moment I get home, I'll take care of all the bills. And by the way, where is yours? You have taken such good care of me that paying you is very much on my mind!" Maybe I was a little reassured for all of us by this seemingly benign statement, but I had also heard that one quite a few times before, so I was still not too optimistic. The subject was then evidently closed, because he added, "Dr. Berczeller, could you ask a rheumatologist to see me? I have had a little pain in my wrist for a couple of hours, and I'd like to make sure that there is nothing to worry about." Up to this point, I had bet my time and that of my consultants on a very questionable risk. I thought, What the hell, we're all so deep in this anyway, and went out to call what was easily the tenth consultation on this never-ending case.

Unfortunately, my suspicions were, even if I can't say "on the money," certainly on the button. Mr. Sherman went home, and none of us ever saw him again. After a while, the bills came back with "Moved, no forwarding address" stamped on them. One day, I did get a letter from him, though. It was very thin (no check in the mail, I thought) and contained a release for his records, which were to be sent to a doctor in Miami. Mr. Sherman was alive! I did not know if he was well in addition, but it was obvious that another doctor had been added to Mr. Sherman's personal, private, socialized medicine scheme.

What Mr. Sherman did was not just run out on a fee for an office visit, which is something like a pickpocketing. Instead, I felt that, in his case, my knowledge and my time had both been looted, like what happens to a store during a riot. What's more, I had been foolish because, although I had been suspicious, I had left the door wide open. Yet I had done the right thing, because, money or not, I had not compromised my standards and had continued to take care of a sick patient. Still, my over-whelming feeling was anger at being used, and I also felt guilty because I had dragged my colleagues into this no-win situation. I had one consolation, though, if only a meager one, and that was the number of times I had been asked to consult on one of *their* deadbeats!

Money

What about the patients who feel they did not get their money's worth from a doctor who seems to them ignorant, negligent, or incompetent, or who just does not seem to care? Certainly many of them do not fall into the category of those who use this kind of complaint as a ploy for the sake of lowering the fee. What's more, they cannot all be wrong, because we know very well that there are doctors who fit these descriptions. Still, there are any number of complaints against doctors that are not at all justified. They arise because patients do not understand that we cannot guarantee results. Medicine is not an exact science like chemistry or physics. As a matter of fact, it is not a science at all. It has a scientific basis, and it is built on anatomy, biochemistry, physiology, microbiology, and the like, which are to a large extent predictable. But an individual body, not to speak of the mind that is attached to it, responds individually to disease, to medication, to the environment. I cannot tell exactly when it is going to die; sometimes, even with the best of intentions, I cannot tell why its condition has unexpectedly improved or worsened. Patients frequently attempt to use the withholding of payment as a bludgeon to punish us for this uncertainty of ours, which looks to them like the ignorance and negligence I mentioned before. They, of course, would like us to guarantee results, and this is why they do not accept our belief that to do so would make us dishonest as well as guilty of falsely playing God.

The only thing we have to sell, or that we have ever had to sell (it is to be hoped that at some time in the future we can say "give"), is our desire to do our very best. This best includes good training, accessibility, a warm link with other human beings, and most important, a great respect for life. Not every doctor deserves high grades in every one of these departments, but the fact that so many of us honestly at least try to do our very best should count in our favor.

More and more of us are beginning to understand that we must look deeper into patients' lives, beyond the obvious illnesses we are asked to treat. Our patients have found a voice and are telling us, more and more frankly, what it is that they don't like about us. In the process, they are telling us much more about themselves than we ever knew. We doctors, on the other hand, have always preferred to suffer in silence and to obtain emotional satisfaction by feeling both virtuous and misunderstood. This may have worked well at a time when patients were a cowed, nonvocal group, but it certainly is to our disadvantage now. We must give them insight into what we do, how long it takes for us to do it, and our own conflicted feelings about being paid for services that go way beyond money in their significance. Otherwise, this sniping about who did what and for whom, and how much it is "worth," will never end.

4

Sex

THE THOUGHT OF a perfect stranger undressing for you is infinitely fascinating for nonphysicians and high on the list of cocktail party conversational gambits when there is a doctor present. What usually happens is that someone pulls you aside and, in a "just us guys" confidential tone, will say, "Sure, you couldn't care less if you are examining some seventy-five-year-old lady, but don't you get *hot* if the patient is some thirty-year-old babe?" The response is not an easy one, even given the fact that the question is not really a question but, rather, a thinly disguised fantasy. Yet the interchange touches a tender spot for me and for all physicians. We know that it is forbidden to take advantage of patients and their dependency on us, but we all worry, at some time or other, whether we can withstand the temptation or the compulsion of the moment. For instance, who will know if you examine the breasts of an especially voluptuous patient one extra, unnecessary time for your own enjoyment? And if a doctor gets a special kick out of having sexually explicit conversations with women, can't he always claim that a particular dialogue was for the sake of delving into the possibly psychosomatic nature of a patient's problem? And, worse yet, what if you are faced with a patient who embodies the last, irresistible missing link in your own sexual fantasies? How can you be sure that you won't lose your head, "just this once," and get involved in a situation that, depending on the outcome, can be defined with words ranging anywhere from *harassment* to *affair*?

Thinking about sex is the favorite pastime of so many people, and doctors are certainly no strangers to this pursuit. As everyone knows, sexual thoughts are not controllable, nor can they be turned off at will. What's more, they pop up at the oddest times and are notoriously terribly distracting. Therefore, I don't consider it at all unusual to have had a sexual reaction to some of my female patients. This reaction was visceral and of the kind I might well have experienced at a party, at a meeting, or while walking on the street. In other words, it was no different from the primitive sexual response we are all prone to, whatever our occupation. But what is interesting, in my case at least, and cocktail party notions aside, is that my sense of being drawn to the patient clicked in as soon as I saw her, *before* I examined her or saw her undressed. Because of this, it seems to me that this sensation is completely instinctive and, as far as I can see, bypasses the intellect. The fact that our fantasies zero in—automatically, it seems—on one object and not on another (the notorious "mental undressing") has forever been the stuff of literature and continues to be a puzzle for all of us in our everyday internal lives.

Irrational attraction is, of course, not a one-way street, and what goes for the doctor also goes for the patient. But if, as it ideally should, sexual magnetism is left at just that on both sides and no attempt is made to act on it, then it can heighten the sympathy and warmth that is absolutely essential for a humane, and not just an impersonal, doctor-patient relationship.

Yet why should doctors not be entitled to swim in the mainstream of sexuality? Are we not as free as any civilian (an endearing term often used by our little special interest group to mean the rest of humanity) to follow up, if we wish, on our impulses? The answer is two times yes, but we can never wriggle out of one overpowering exception, and it is this: In our dealings with patients, while thinking about sex is unavoidable and basically harmless, any attempt on our part to act out these fantasies is not only immoral and completely against our code of professional conduct but can also cause grave psychological harm to the very people whom we are obligated to protect, our patients.

Happily, most of us have a built-in mechanism that prevents us from any expression of our sexual feelings toward patients. Call it a taboo, something deeply ingrained within us, and not just a vague response to one of a list of no-no's learned in a long-ago ethics course. Are all doctors subject to this taboo? Evidently not, but that does not mean that these exceptions to the norm are all sex abusers. It is, rather, that when they are faced with sexual feelings for patients, these doctors have to make a case-by-case moral decision, which is something that can be not only emotionally very draining but also full of unforeseen dangers.

I was twenty-three years old, and at the end of my sophomore year in medical school, when I first encountered this powerful fail-safe switch within myself. It was in the physical diagnosis course, where we were learning how to examine patients. After having done thousands of physical examinations over the years, it is difficult for me to imagine now that there was a time in my life when I did not possess the special skills of vision, touch, hearing, smell, and judgment that are so much a part of me now. But at that point, after several hours of lectures, and after we had learned to take blood pressures on each other, my class was divided into groups of two and each team was assigned to an individual patient on Ward 64, the largest female ward at Chicago's Cook County Hospital. Most of us had never been "upstairs" on the wards, which smelled mainly of disinfectant with a touch of the odors of stool and urine thrown in, but at least the hospital was not completely unfamiliar to us, since we had already attended some lectures in its ancient, ill-lit amphitheaters, which went back to the nineteenth century.

A few of us walked up the stairs gingerly holding brand-new doctors' bags with our names imprinted on them in gold letters (courtesy of a drug company); I know we must have looked like scared children on the way to the principal's office. As Phil Stone, my partner, and I climbed the stairs as slowly as we could, trying to put off the coming ordeal for as long as possible, we chattered nervously about who K. Gorczynski (that was the name of "our" patient) could possibly be. What's more, especially since we were also expected to take a history, might we not have the misfortune of having to examine someone who did not speak English, only Polish?

In the 1950s, and especially in so-called charity hospitals like Cook County, there was much less regard for the patients' privacy than there is nowadays. At that time, curtains that could be drawn around each bed were still something in the future, but we had heard through the grapevine that the ward was equipped with a few movable screens on wheels. I wish I could say that we were concerned with protecting our patient from embarrassment, but my associate and I had agreed beforehand that we would place as many screens as possible around her bed in order to hide our obvious ineptness from the staff as well as from other patients, who, we had heard, were not at all reluctant to offer embarrassingly graphic critiques of the skills of students and residents alike, and not too quietly either.

The two screens we had found were squeaking as we dragged them along the linoleum-covered, littered floor of the ward. We stopped at the assigned bed, number 15. A young blond woman of about twenty was sitting on it, her dangling feet accentuated by toenails painted a bright red. She was wearing what appeared to be general-issue hospital pajamas, but what set her off from the dirty beige wall behind her was a bandanna tied around her waist. It was of exactly the same shade as her toenails, and—as a bonus, it seemed to me—it helped to show her obviously large breasts to good advantage. When my partner asked her, in an unfamiliar, strangled voice, whether she indeed was K. Gorczynski, and she, in lightly accented but excellent English, admitted smilingly that she was, my first reaction was one of joy. Far from the ordeal of being forced to deal with some uncooperative, decrepit old lady, which is what I had expected, I (my partner's existence had suddenly been erased from my mind) was going to be lucky enough to be able to examine, as thoroughly as I knew how, this friendly, pretty, buxom woman.

After taking her history (she had had pneumonia), we began our examination. We stood to each side of her and began with what we knew best, taking the blood pressure. As soon as we started, she began to blush in a shade not that different from the toenails and the bandanna that were now totally hidden under the sheet with which we had fastidiously covered her from the neck down. She had a right to be embarrassed. After all, we must really have been just boys in her eyes, and of approximately her own age, to boot. For a moment I wanted very badly to run away, to leave all this medical stuff to adults. I didn't, of course, and it was not because of any great professionalism on my part but because the examination itself had begun to take on a life of its own. My participation was clearly essential, and so was Phil's, not to speak of the young girl's. She had, involuntarily and by complete accident, become involved in this attempt to teach us our trade.

So we continued, and Phil and I each checked one eye and one ear, joined forces for the one thyroid and throat, and finally arrived at the breasts. As we stood there, one of us examining the right breast and the other the left, with the patient seemingly suspended between our four hands, we all looked at one another and burst out laughing. It must really have been a funny scene, and we knew it. When we finally stopped, the ice had been broken, we all relaxed, and the rest of the exercise went more smoothly than we could have hoped. Yet my embarrassment (as well as pity) for her, my initial sexual arousal, and the sense of release that I felt from the perception of how ridiculous we looked, merged with the realization that I was *actually* in a hospital and examining a patient. These potent impressions and emotions, coming together in some mysterious interaction, must have triggered my first real, adult understanding of the seriousness of not only what we were doing then but also of what we were going to be doing in the future, after we became doctors. Most of us can only recognize critical moments in our lives by looking back upon them, and sometimes, for reasons that are not clear, we produce the memory of a critical moment when, actually, the change was just gradual. But I can pinpoint that tiny segment of time, just after we stopped laughing, when my still-adolescent fantasies about sex gave way to the inhibitions of professional thinking and behavior. This is why I have never forgotten the patient's name or her bed number. The encounter with K. Gorczynski of bed 15 still is for me an unforgettable part of the process of what our dean, John Sheinin, used to call "turning a boy into a doctor."

But then again, being the owner of such a vital taboo does not guarantee that it will not be tested from time to time. This happened to me only a few years after the episode at Cook County Hospital. I was then a third-year resident in internal medicine and used to make house calls in my free time. Trainees' salaries were piteously low in the 1950s, and I needed the outside money not only for my daily expenses but also to pay the installments on a gleaming black Plymouth convertible I had recently bought in a fit of impetuous optimism. My busy schedule would have kept me from the social life of a normal twenty-six-year-old if I had not had the idea (forced by circumstance) of combining moonlighting and dates. So it was not unusual that I had company as I drove toward the St. Regis, a luxury hotel in mid-Manhattan where I had been called to see a patient. It was a sunny June afternoon, the top was down, and I remember how lucky I felt. Not only was my girlfriend, Barbara, a tall brunette with an upswept hairdo, high cheek-bones, and beautiful green eyes, sitting next to me, I was also young, a doctor, and even making a little money. I still remember it as one of those especially happy, memorable days, and it was to be capped with dinner at Ruc, a Czech restaurant on Seventy-second Street, where the attraction of the roast duck, dumplings, and cold draft beer was exceeded only by the charm of the backyard garden setting with its red-bedecked tables and old trees festooned with strings of multicolored lights.

The patient received me in the living room of what was obviously a luxury suite. On first glance, she did not seem to be particularly ill. Judging from her accent, there was no question that she was French, and she volunteered the information that she was the executive secretary of one of the most important movie producers of that time.

She was of medium height and had reddish blond hair that she wore loose. Although she was fully dressed, it was evident that she had a magnificent body, and her voice had a low-pitched, smoky quality. As soon as I saw her, I lost whatever professional manner I had managed to acquire by that time. To my relief, her only complaint was a sore throat. As I approached to examine her, I entered the magnetic field of her perfume, which smelled like a whole garden of exotic flowers. This made me so confused that, when I put a tongue depressor into her mouth, I saw nothing at all at first; I had forgotten to turn on the flashlight! Subsequently, I made a major blunder when I listened to the chest through her deep yellow cashmere sweater (exposing the area to be examined is a basic rule in physical diagnosis and one that every second-year medical student already follows). I then gave her a prescription for an antibiotic, forgot to collect my fee, and finally escaped after suggesting that, by the next morning, she call the person for whom I was covering.

When I came out onto the street, the weather was still balmy, the car still shiny, and Barbara as beautiful as ever. But it was I who had changed. I had been completely transfixed by my patient and could not stop thinking about her. The dinner that night was a failure. I was distracted, which in turn made Barbara angry, and the end of the day completely betrayed the promise of its beginning.

Over the next several days, I continued to regret my immature behavior toward the French lady at the St. Regis, as well as my inability to ask her out because, however brief the encounter, she was at least technically my patient. But on the morning of the third day, she called me at the hospital. I do not know how she found me, since I had neither office nor answering service, but she was very definite about wanting to see me "not as a patient." I tried to explain my conflict as well as I could. Still, she insisted. She was leaving for France shortly, and while she understood my objections very well, she still wanted to have dinner with me. I did not know what to do. I was tempted, yes, but I also felt uneasy. I did not want to be discourteous, but what finally tipped the balance was that voice, which brought her presence and her scent back to me, and I finally agreed.

We went out that same evening, and I was, if it was possible, even more mesmerized by her than before. But I was too ambivalent, and as the evening wore on, I became more and more withdrawn. I guess I must have expected to be struck down at any moment by the particular lightning reserved for young doctors with questionable ethics, and I acted accordingly. Finally, she gave up. She complained of a sudden return of her sore throat but did not ask me to reexamine her. I soon took her back to her hotel, and we shook hands, as patient and doctor usually do when they say good-bye.

Of course, I have thought about this incident over the years. At times I am sorry that I could not enjoy the moment, that I did not engage in a small adventure with an especially attractive woman with whom my professional contact had, after all, been minimal. Much of the time, though, I am in sympathy with my younger self. I must have understoood then what I still know now, that when a doctor and his patient engage in a sexual relationship, the roles of the partners are far from equal. The patient's motives can well be multiple, ranging from love to money, by way of hero worship, but her moral being is not affected by the affair. The doctor, on the other hand, automatically violates his patient's trust in this situation and is morally and professionally diminished as well.

By a narrow margin, I made a choice that robbed me of a memorable encounter. I still believe that what I did was right, but how I sometimes wish I had met her *before* encountering K. Gorczynski in that course at Cook County Hospital!

It can be very difficult to draw the line between the friendly attentions of a physically demonstrative doctor and frank sexual overtures. But even if there is no question about it, and it is perfectly obvious that something sexual and not just medical is going on, patients often fear to come forward. A woman in this situation is usually afraid of "blowing the whistle" because she does not want to be disapproved of, or dismissed by, somebody important to her—for instance, the man who delivered her children. But she knows that something that should not have happened did happen, and she is in a terrible bind. Ultimately, she may either deny the entire episode, falsely blame herself for being "paranoid," and stay with the doctor, or she may leave him. If something undeniable such as actual intercourse has taken place, rationalization is, of course, much more difficult. But even then, women often keep quiet because, although they are blameless, they are too ashamed of what has happened and do not want anyone to know about it.

I was personally faced with a problem of this kind early on in my career. When my wife became pregnant with our first child, we decided as a matter of course to ask the chief of obstetrics and gynecology at what was then my principal hospital to undertake her care. My wife had known him since her student nurse days, and I had come to respect his skill highly ever since my rotation on his service during my internship. What's more, we had encountered him and his family by chance during our honeymoon in Acapulco and since that time had had social contact with him as well. At a party or at a dinner, he was invariably both paternal and charming, so that, all in all, he appeared to be an ideal choice for us.

Yet, one day late in her second trimester, my wife called me at my office, something she rarely did. She was highly upset, and since I knew that she had been to see the "Big Chief" (as everyone called him, not only because of his rank but also because of his girth) for a routine prenatal visit, I at first thought that something had gone wrong with the pregnancy.

She was able to tell me that she and the baby were fine, but she sounded so agitated that I ran across the street to our apartment as soon as I had finished seeing my patient.

My wife, who has always set a standard of calmness for our otherwise temperamental family, was crying and pacing up and down the room. She was pale, her hands were cold, and it was only with some difficulty that I persuaded her to lie down on the couch and allow me to cover her with a blanket. Then the story came out. Toward the end of the examination, the "Big Chief" had abruptly sent his nurse out of the examining room. He then put his arms around my wife and tried to kiss her, all the while murmuring how much he loved pregnant women. My wife remembered being stunned, but she had had the presence of mind to ask him to leave the room. She then got dressed and simply walked out of the office.

By this time, taking a careful history had become second nature to me, and I began to quiz her very thoroughly about what had happened. I freely admit that I was hoping all the while that it had been a big misunderstanding and that she had mistaken her doctor's usual friendliness for a sexual advance. But deep down, I knew that she was not given to hysterical misjudgments. As my wife began to calm down, I became more and more angry. The "Big Chief" had assaulted my wife and violated our trust, and my anger was, if anything, more intense because he was a fellow doctor. As a matter of fact, I began to have visions that evening of going to his office, punching him in the nose, and then denouncing him to the medical board of the hospital. Like any other husband, doctor or not, I tried to console my wife as well as I could. We never slept that night, and we went over the event again and again and again—as do, for instance, survivors of a car wreck or a plane crash.

My wife's face and voice became sadder as we talked. I tried to cheer her up with empty optimism (nothing *really* happened, and so on), but she quickly interrupted my nervous chattering and began to explain to me how much she thought she had lost. The chief's actions had not only wounded and frightened her, they had also violently interrupted the peaceful progress of her pregnancy. We would now be in the uncomfortable position of shopping around for another doctor when she was already in her sixth month. What would we give as the reason for leaving the chief and going to someone else in his department? In my concern and anger, I had not even considered these practical questions, but what she expressed next was completely unexpected. Wistfully, she began to tell me how much she would miss her doctor's reassuring smile and warm manner, and how very sorry she was that her relationship with him had to end this way. Her nostalgia made me jealous. How could she be mourning for a relationship with someone who had attempted such a low trick? We had, of course, agreed from the beginning that we would go to another doctor, but I began to realize that her ambivalent feelings toward the chief would not be resolved nearly as quickly as the choice of his replacement. In this way I learned at first hand how tight the bond between patient and doctor in obstetrics really is and how much it takes to rupture it.

Like most others in this predicament, we did not pursue the punishment of the doctor. We could not prove that anything had really happened, it would be his word against my wife's, and so on. Unlike most others, however, I had a special problem. I was only a junior doctor in a hospital where the "Big Chief" was politically powerful, so I knew that our blowing the whistle on him would, whatever the ultimate outcome, bring the wrath of the hospital hierarchy down on my head.

I think about this incident sometimes (more often than one would think after a lapse of thirty years), and I am still angry with him and disappointed with myself. Career or no, should I not have punched him in the nose and for good measure gone public with our accusation? My wife suffered unnecessarily during what should have been a golden time for her: the upcoming birth of her first child. The doctor should have been punished for her suffering, but instead I let him off the hook. Whether what he did to my wife was part of a pattern or a one-time occurrence is still not clear. Yet we will always be left with an unpleasant memory that intrudes on the happy memories of the birth of our firstborn. What's more, I have a personal bonus to show for this sorry affair: guilt for letting my own career ambitions interfere with what should have been my first priority, protecting my wife.

What happened to us is not unique. There is no question about the fact that doctors abuse patients sexually, and I will describe more instances of this abuse a little later. The public is suspicious, sometimes for very good reason, that doctors "cover up" for each other. I certainly have no intention of doing that, and as a matter of fact, I deplore the uneven self-policing of our profession, which can only result in diminished trust in all of us.

On the other hand, though, the unusual nature of the every-day contact between doctors and patients has to be considered before the guilt of all doctors faced with sexually related charges is taken for granted. For example, in trying to make a diagnosis, I am completely justified in asking what seem to be highly intimate questions that often do not seem relevant to the patient. If I inquire about the recency and frequency of oral sex, a young woman with a persistent sore throat may well feel offended. Yet I must at least consider upper respiratory tract gonorrhea as a cause of her symptoms, so that it is my obliga-tion to ask.

As another example, we routinely consider the entire body to be open territory when we search for physical findings that could help in clarifying the diagnosis of a complicated illness. Specifically focusing on the size of the clitoris, for example, may well appear to a patient to be too drastic an invasion of her pri-vacy. Did she only hear (but not necessarily understand) my explanation of the connection between an overactive adrenal gland and enlargement of this sexually significant organ?

Because we constantly play this game of show-and-tell with our patients, we are always at risk for having our motives misinterpreted. Yet how does a doctor avoid a "bum rap" and still continue to provide good patient care without constantly being afraid? It seems that good luck has something to do with it, but then again, so does professional behavior that is appropriate to the situation and that at all times maintains the dignity of both patient and doctor. Lots of doctors give a kiss on the cheek to some of their female patients when they say hello and goodbye, for example, and I am certainly one of them. But there is a vast difference between this spontaneous and friendly act that can be compared to a handshake and, for instance, adding a sexually suggestive remark to the kiss. The telling of "dirty" jokes, the recounting of one's own sexual exploits, and open admiration of a patient's physical attractiveness are also maneuvers the experienced doctor avoids at all costs.

On the other hand, patients have very good instincts. Most of the time they know very well whom to trust, and this extends to sexual matters as well. If a doctor (and his office) are consistent in creating an atmosphere of "all business"—combined, of course, with evident concern and a desire to be of help—it is much less likely that misunderstandings about sexual behavior will arise.

Medicine, God knows, is not exempt from Murphy's law. As a matter of fact, and especially if we take into account the unpredictable nature of what we do, if anything can go wrong, it will go wrong. Besides, we ourselves are only human, and patients think and do the damnedest things. Regardless of the large numbers of patients who go into the statistics so irreplaceable for health policy experts, the best medicine still resolves down to one doctor and one patient alone in a room. In this setting, confidentiality is preserved, the patient's sense of privacy is reinforced, and it is to be hoped that he (not necessarily always, I am sad to admit) has the doctor's entire attention. Unfortunately, though, the examining room sometimes turns into a lion's cage when either patient or doctor has a hidden sexual agenda; then the roles of the lion and the Christian are assumed accordingly.

I will never forget the case of Frank, a friend of my father's who practiced on Seventy-ninth Street in Manhattan in what was then a Hungarian neighborhood. He had been called Ferenc in the old country but had proudly anglicized his name when he arrived here. Like my father and many general practitioners of the time, he worked alone in his office, answering the telephone, doing his own electrocardiograms, and so on. One evening, while my father and I were toting up the day's receipts (I was his confidential though unpaid secretary), Frank came into our combination office-apartment unannounced. Even before he began to speak, I could sense that there was something wrong. Frank's usually carefully combed hair was disarranged, and his face had a reddish color I had never seen before. Besides, he must have left his office in a hurry, since he was still in his white lab coat. There was none of the customary elaborate greeting to me in Hungarian (the joke had always been, of course, that I could not speak Hungarian) but, rather, the urgent telling of what was evidently a story in the same language. My always cheerful father began to look more and more troubled as he listened to what Frank was telling him, and I was soon sent out of the room. My dismissal puzzled me. After all, I could not understand what they were saying anyway. I expected my curiosity to be satisfied as soon as I could speak to my father alone, so I took up a watch in the empty waiting room and waited for Frank to leave. But when I was called back into the combination consulting and examining room after Frank's departure, I was able to get very little information, although I asked a lot of questions. I was really very surprised, because my father had always been very open with me, and I had already acquired a precocious knowledge of such diverse subjects as his first love, his first Fascist jail, and so on. "When you are a doctor, don't ever do an internal examination on a woman without another woman present" was the only thing he was willing to say, with great emphasis on *ever* and *another*. Then he added, "Why do you think I always call your mother in, even if she is busy cooking next door, when I am ready to do a pelvic?" I was sixteen years old and had already been given to understand that I was expected to become a doctor (letting people make their own career decisions was not my family's strong suit), but the question of what to do about a particular examination was absolutely of no interest to me.

Yet I continued to wonder, off and on, what they had talked about in the office and what the big mystery was all about. Years later, when I was in medical school, Frank died, and then my father told me the whole story. A new patient, a young woman, had come to see Frank complaining of vaginal bleeding. After he had set her up in stirrups and was preparing to put a speculum into her vagina, she suddenly jumped off the examining table and, in an ever louder voice, claimed that he had tried to rape her. Frank tried to calm her down, saying that he hadn't even started to examine her yet, and asked her to lower her voice since there were patients in the waiting room. She immediately quieted down and then proposed a deal. Instead of going to the police and exposing his "shameful" conduct, she demanded one hundred dollars then and fifty dollars a week (this happened in the 1940s) in return for the "ordeal" she had gone through. Frank went along with the bargain, not only because he did not want to lose his up to then good medical reputation but also because, as a relatively recent immigrant, he was afraid of possible problems with the law of his adoptive country. Although he could have called the woman's bluff, no one can blame him for his decision. The stakes were just too high for him. As it happened, his blackmailer came back for three or four installments and then disappeared. Fortunately, he never saw her again.

Frank's story (and although no one can vouch for his version, I believe it to this day) has always stayed with me. I have thought about it from time to time, and it has made me wonder how a doctor can protect himself not only against a blackmailer but also from the unwanted attentions of a woman who, for whatever reasons of her own, wants to have sex with him. He is in a bind, because if he refuses, the woman may, out of anger, claim that it was he who initiated the advances. A doctor's reputation is a very fragile thing. The slightest question about it, the merest rumor about his sexual interest in patients, even if he is completely innocent of the accusations leveled against him, can harm him for the rest of his professional life. Although his colleagues may vouch for him, and even if a board of professional misconduct exonerates him, the question of his guilt is likely to remain in the minds of his patients and his community. Yet we Americans rightly put great emphasis on the principle that a person is innocent until proven guilty. Then why should doctors, whose livelihood, professional standing, and peace of mind are at risk every time someone levels an accusation against them, with whatever justification, not enjoy the same privilege as the society that is made up of their patients?

I had one near-accident a few years after I went into practice. I had seen a sixteen-year-old girl for the first time, on a house call, and made a diagnosis of infectious mononucleosis. I remember thinking at the time that she looked more mature than sixteen, and also not only that she was quite buxom but that her manner was unusually coquettish for someone of that age. Teenage girls, in my experience, tend to be sullen and withdrawn when meeting a strange doctor. My patient, on the other hand, spoke and laughed a lot and competed very openly for my attention with her mother. What's more, she wore the shortest shorty pajamas I had ever encountered and positioned herself on the sickbed in several poses that must have been suggested to her by a thorough study of a *Playboy* centerfold. After writing out a prescription for relief of her sore throat (there was then, and still is, no specific treatment for infectious mononucleosis), I suggested that she see me a few days later for a blood test and follow-up examination.

Since I had an unbreakable office rule that all female patients under eighteen had to be accompanied by a female relative, I expected the girl's mother to be there on the day of the appointment. Yet when I went in to see the girl in one of my examining rooms, I noticed that the paper gown that must have been offered to her was lying unused on the floor. My precocious patient was reclining on the examining table on her side and facing the door, her chin cradled in one of her palms. She was completely naked, and the whole scene bore a resemblance, this time, not to seductive poses learned in magazines but to Velazquez's portrait of the Duchess of Alba, which so shocked the Spanish court centuries ago. I did not enter the room but stopped at the threshold. She said something like "Come in, Doctor, I'm ready," which, under other circumstances and with another patient, might have been a completely innocent statement. What was worse, her mother was nowhere in sight, and the realization immediately came to me that my office staff had somehow been hoodwinked into breaking my below-eighteen rule. I knew instinctively that I was in danger. I could, of course, have called my nurse in to be present during the examination, but I understood that even if I were fortunate enough to avoid disaster on this occasion, I would never stop being at risk if I continued to take care of this sexually aggressive, manipulative child. I did not say a word but instead closed the door. I then asked my nurse to tell the patient to get dressed, go home, and have her mother call me.

My intention was to recommend that she take her daughter back to the family pediatrician, a very capable woman, but I never heard from either mother or daughter again.

For the onlooker, and even in the memory of those who are directly involved, near-disasters do not come close to having the same impact as the real article. Yet even after such a long time, I can easily summon up the dread I felt when I was standing at the door of that examining room—and my sense of relief when that girl was finally dispatched from my office.

Hospitals are like little villages, and everybody knows everything that is going on. This is how, over the years, I heard a few stories of questionable sexual behavior on the part of doctors of my acquaintance. I cannot, of course, vouch for anyone's guilt or innocence, so I report the facts as I heard them. Sex abuse by doctors is no different from that done by anyone else. We have our rapists, our gropers, our self-exposers; in fact, we have the entire range of sexual offenders. What is different, though, is that patients present themselves trustingly to these psychiatrically disturbed physicians, who do not even have to go searching for victims. Working under the umbrella of "normal" medical activities, these doctors create even more harm by raising doubts in their patients' minds about the appropriateness (and propriety) of what they are doing.

Psychiatric illness may be less obvious to the onlooker, but it is no less devastating than cancer or severe heart disease. The story of someone I will call Larry is a tragic example of disturbed sexual behavior in a physician. He was an acknowledged star at an early age. While still in his thirties, he did fine research that ended up in the original description of a new disease. What's more, he was an excellent clinician with a large practice, and he was also a popular and respected teacher. My shock may be understandable, then, when I heard through the usually reliable hospital grapevine, a few years ago, that Larry had just had his license suspended. It was almost as dramatic as if I had heard that he had died, so I immediately began to call around to find out what had happened. The best that I could find out at the time was that not only one but a few of his female patients had complained to a state agency about sexual abuse at Larry's hands. Even my best-informed sources, though, the ones who usually knew all the secrets of hospital life, did not know what it was exactly that Larry was supposed to have done. The only thing they knew was that, after a hearing, the agency had decided to temporarily lift his right to practice pending psychiatric therapy.

I could not avoid wondering about it. Was he a groper, someone who let his hands wander inappropriately around the bodies of some of the women under his care? Was he a rapist? Was he a flasher? As it turned out, I only got an insight into Larry's special tendencies more than a year later, after he came back into practice, his license having been restored. For several months after his return, whenever I met him in the hospital, he invariably looked his usual elegant self, and what's more, he acted as if he had just come back from some prestigious sabbatical and not from the suspension of his license. And then he suddenly disappeared again. This time, the events leading up to the permanent loss of his license were better known. He was evidently a groper after all, and his latest problem had come up after the mother of one of his young patients in the clinic had complained to the hospital administration that he had attempted to caress her while she was there as a chaperone for her daughter.

New York is a very large city, mercifully so when you don't want to bump into someone. To avoid the inevitable embarrassment, I would have been just as glad never to see Larry again.

Yet, a few months after he left the hospital for good, I did see him in a well-known bookstore on Madison Avenue where I occasionally go to browse on Saturday afternoons. What struck me first was that, unlike the other clerks in their unisex outfits of jeans and open-necked shirts, the man transacting a sale at the computer was unusually well dressed. I knew that he was not the owner of the store, and then I realized almost immediately that it was Larry at the counter, in a double-breasted suit, white shirt, probably a Hermes tie, and a handkerchief in his breast pocket. As a matter of fact, he seemed almost unchanged from the way he had always looked in the doctors' coatroom at the hospital as he was preparing to make rounds. I say "almost" because there was one thing missing, and that was the red-tubed stethoscope, his famous trademark, which the old Larry had always carried slung around his neck.

At that moment, I felt terribly sad for him, although he had never been more than a hospital acquaintance of mine and I had been only a distant witness to his tragedy. Did I think that he had been unfairly treated? No, not at all. Considering the number of complaints and the two separate series of incidents, it was very unlikely that he was innocent of the accusations made against him. Was the punishment too strong? No. I certainly did not feel differently then than I do now, and I believe that a physician who is sexually aggressive toward patients, and especially when that behavior has not been changed by psychotherapy, should not be allowed to practice. But seeing him there, still looking very much the doctor but reduced to making a living as a salesclerk, made me very unhappy. His psychiatric illness had obviously given him no rest and his innocent patients were tortured unnecessarily, and in the meantime, he had done something irrevocable—he had committed professional suicide.

As soon as I saw him, I turned around quickly, hoping that he had not noticed me. Fortunately, the store was crowded and

I was able to escape, heart racing and suddenly perspiring as if it had been July and not a cold December day.

But why the alarm reaction, the beating heart, the sense of panic? I think it had more to do with the rest of us than with Larry. At that moment, it must have been more clear to me than ever before what a tightrope we doctors walk and how illness, absence of taboo, a hostile patient, just a plain accident, or any combination of all of these was capable of pushing any of us to the counter of that bookstore. Certainly I did (and still do) have sympathy for both Larry and the people he frightened and confused. But I was also very grateful that I was not in his shoes. It seems to me now that the collision between pity and relief caused the anxiety and agitation I was feeling. I admit it! I have very little courage for this kind of thing, and if I were ever to see Larry again, I would probably have the same reaction all over again. In the meantime, just to make sure, I am doing my Saturday book browsing in a different part of town.

Into what category do you put doctors who marry their patients? Do you look under *A*, for abuse, or under *L*, for love? Just because the encounter ends up in marriage, does that excuse a sexual relationship between patient and doctor? I had never even considered these questions until about twenty-five years ago. At that time I was taking care of an English airline stewardess who had a puzzling combination of symptoms. She had repeated rashes, fevers, and joint pains, and despite an elaborate and expensive investigation, as well as many curbstone consultations with my colleagues, I could not come up with an answer to her problem. At that point, I thought it was only fair to refer her to one of the respected older subspecialists in my department for a formal second opinion. Over the next few days, I waited impatiently for his findings while personally suffering from equal doses of frustration and curiosity. Second opinions are often not much better than first ones, and as it turned out, he did not have much to add. He praised me for my workup, suggested several more tests (par for the course), and referred the patient back to me. I was flattered by his vote of confidence, and by now I was more than ever intrigued by the patient's unusual illness. But my enigmatic stewardess never came back, and what's more, she did not respond to several calls from my secretary. I could not understand what had gone wrong between us. After all, I had done my best to find out what was wrong with her, and we had always gotten along very well. I was hurt and puzzled, but several months later I suddenly understood everything when a casual scanning of the wedding announcements in the *New York Times* revealed to me that my patient and my consultant had just been married!

Since that time, the same questions come up in my mind whenever I see this couple at a medical center social event. What did her diagnosis turn out to be? I don't think I will ever know, but maybe her husband finally came up with an answer. The more piquant question, though, is what really happened with them at the beginning and at what point did their relationship change? Was it sex first? If so, initiated by which one? Or was the consultation like a blind date, but with love at first sight and sex as a sequel?

Of course, I do not expect to find out the answers to these questions, either. But the whole issue raises other problems in my mind. For instance, if a doctor falls in love with a patient, and if his feelings are reciprocated, is it immoral under these circumstances to consider marriage? Or if a doctor and patient find each other to be sexually irresistible, is it "permissible" for him to enter into a relationship if he first sends her for further care to another physician? Or is it ethical (and this happened to a doctor friend of mine) for a pediatrician to have an affair with the mother of one of his little patients?

These are borderline situations that point out the ambiguous links some of us have with our patients. Is there a right and wrong in these cases? Sometimes there is, but sometimes they are just too close to call. It is especially these problematic detours in people's lives that most deserve our patience and understanding, because they involve something that does not come along all that frequently and that should therefore not be minimized, and that is a chance for happiness.

5

Are Families Good for You?

ASK ANY DOCTOR how he feels about patients' families. If he is being honest and not just keeping his emotions to himself, as we oftem do, he will have many stories to tell about interference by relatives and how this made his job of taking care of the patient much more difficult. But he will very likely also reminisce about the families who gave him leeway to do what he had to while, at the same time, they stayed close and available, so that they gave comfort not only to the patient but to him as well.

I am no different from my colleagues in this respect. Yet stories about helpful, reassuring, and cooperative relatives tend to get lost in the shuffle of what seems to be the greater number of unpleasant experiences with members of patients' families. I admit that it is difficult not to lose your head when someone close to you is very sick. Yet if a family can maintain its poise in this situation, and I admit that it takes great effort, the result will be a much more constructive relationship with the doctor. He will then be able to concentrate fully on the medical problems of the patient without the distraction of having to defend himself, for instance, against that favorite maneuver: finding a scapegoat if things do not work out with the patient as they are supposed to.

I first saw Howard Kalb late one evening. His mother had

called a family friend, a podiatrist who had his office next to mine, for a referral to an internist, and he suggested that she call me. As she was describing her son's symptoms, though, I became alarmed enough to decide not to wait until the next morning to see him, and asked her to bring him right over to the emergency room.

He was eighteen years old at the time (this was a few years ago) and had been well until several days before, when he began to have numbness of his feet. Since that time he had had increasing weakness of his muscles, and earlier in the evening that I saw him, he had found that he could no longer take a deep breath because of weakness of his chest muscles.

It had sounded like Guillain-Barré syndrome to me over the telephone, and when I saw him I found no reason to change my original impression. His poor reflexes and droopy upper eyelids (due to weakness of the lid muscles) helped to confirm my preliminary diagnosis. Over the years, I had seen a few patients with this condition, which is probably caused by a virus and sometimes accompanies mononucleosis. These people are usually young and otherwise healthy, and almost always recover completely within weeks to months. They are liable to go into respiratory failure, though; in other words, they may have severe breathing difficulties, and as a matter of fact, the first Guillain-Barré patient I ever saw, in 1955, required an iron lung until her own chest muscles began to function normally again.

I personally cannot imagine being a pediatrician. What I mean to say is that taking responsibility for the health and life of a small child is something I consider too much to bear emotionally. Yet pediatricians thrive on the security of knowing that *most* of their patients are healthy, and they, in turn, cannot imagine taking care of adults, who are much more likely to be seriously ill and who can easily die in the process. Teenagers are still children as far as I am concerned, but, usually in response to requests by their parents, I used to start seeing what are called young adults, after the age of sixteen or seventeen.

Of course, I had to have come to grips with illness and death in adults, otherwise I could not have done what I did. But facing these possibilities in patients who belong in that no-man's-land between childhood and adulthood has always made me very uncomfortable, so I saw as few of them as possible.

That evening, I was preparing myself for the possibility of having to deal with hysterical parents, especially since I had found out from Howard that he was an only child. I have two sons who were in his general age group when I began to take care of him, and I have always (even though they are now thirty-one and twenty-seven) tended to be anxious about them. There was not even any question about it. I already had, in advance, a large reservoir of understanding for whatever outrageous behavior his parents might engage in, but I promised myself that nothing would keep me from taking care of this child as if he were my own.

Of course, I should have realized that there was something unusual going on when I had not, as would have been expected, seen his parents hovering over his stretcher in the little cubicle he had been assigned to. It was a momentary observation I made when I first came in and introduced myself to him, and the first thought that came into my mind at the time was an automatic one, which came from my many years of practicing in New York City. It seems that here, every patient has a relative who is a doctor, and if not that, then at least he has a friend whose son-in-law is, for example, a hospital administrator and who "knows the best doctors in town." So I would not have been surprised if the parents had, at that moment, been at the public telephone outside the emergency room, checking out my credentials or possibly even making arrangements to transfer Howard to another recommended hospital.

After securing an intensive care unit bed, ordering further

tests, including a spinal tap and blood gases (his oxygenation was adequate so far), and calling for a neurological consultation, I went looking for his parents. Of course, I did not know what they looked like, but clinicians are well known for their improvising skills, so the first thing I did was to screen the people in the waiting room for a resemblance to Howard. There was no real problem. His mother stood out of the crowd as an older, female Howard; this was Jenny, who was to become a great friend of mine. She was short, stocky, round faced, with blond hair, and spoke with a strong German accent. Howard's father, who was to die under my care just a few months later and was already harboring his cancer of the lung when we first met, was also short and spoke slowly in a low voice. Only later on, when I got to know them better, did I realize that Jenny must always have been in charge of communications for the family and that Herman, her husband, owed his halting way of speech to the fact that—in a sense, like a deaf-mute—he did not often enough hear the sound of his own voice.

When I introduced myself, Jenny immediately gave me a big smile. I was suspicious. Did this woman think that the sick boy inside was a laughing matter? Would I have smiled under these circumstances? Never! I could not even have stopped my pacing up and down long enough to greet the doctor if it had been my child in that cubicle! But the smile was just the beginning, and it preceded her thanks for my agreeing to take care of Howard. I told them what I knew so far: that, if the diagnosis was correct, he would recover with time, but that we would have to watch his breathing very carefully and we should not hesitate to do a tracheostomy (make a hole in his windpipe) to help his breathing if his chest muscles became any weaker. I did not know if they had expected the news to be so serious, and although I noticed that Jenny's smile had faded, they listened without interrupting me. I thought it would be reassuring for them to know that a neurologist would help me in taking care of their son, but to my surprise, she said, "Doctor, whatever you do is fine with us. Our friend Bob [the podiatrist] recommended you highly, and we know this is a wonderful hospital, so do what you have to do, we trust you!" I was amazed by their approach (it seemed that she was, as usual, speaking for both of them), but this vote of confidence, which I had not yet earned, helped me past some of the uncertainty and fear doctors feel so often, especially at the beginning of a difficult case. Things might not be so rosy later on, I thought, but for the moment I was happy just to concentrate on the patient, who needed all the attention I could give him.

It was only several days later, again late in the evening, after Howard's respiratory muscle function had been worsening all day and the muscles in other parts of his body were also becoming weaker, that I got some insight into Jenny's and Herman's remarkable attitude. As we waited for the surgeon who was to do the tracheostomy at the bedside, I voiced some of my doubts to them about my original diagnosis of Guillain-Barré syndrome. Since there is no definitive test for this condition, and because the timetable for the paralysis was turning out not to be typical for it, either, I was beginning to consider several other diagnoses that would fit into the picture that was developing in front of us. I had retaken Howard's history earlier that day, and he had admitted that he had eaten some food out of a can, food that in thinking back had smelled "funny," several days before the beginning of his illness. I brought up the question because I had thought of botulism as another possible cause for his neurological problem. This is a condition that can be confused with Guillain-Barré. In botulism, a toxin poisonous to the nerves is produced by bacteria that grow in putrefying food. An antidote for the toxin was available, so it was obviously important to decide whether he had botulism, which is almost always fatal unless the patient is treated, or Guillain-Barré, which ultimately gets better on its own. The neurologist, an infectious disease specialist I had consulted, and I had decided, later that same day, to stick with the diagnosis of Guillain-Barré, which was still more in keeping with the total clinical picture of the patient. The diagnosis of botulism was not out of the question, but it seemed less likely, especially since at this point most untreated patients with this condition would already have been dead.

It was one of those deceptively calm moments that are occasionally encountered in dealing with critical illnesses, something like floating in the eye of a hurricane. The Kalbs and I were sitting there waiting, as I said, for the surgeon to come out of the operating room. We had already agreed that he was to make a hole in Howard's windpipe so that we could replace, with a positive-pressure machine, the chest muscles that normally drive respiration. I do not know exactly what led up to it, but Jenny started to tell me something of her family's past. I had, of course, correctly guessed that she was German by birth, but I had thought that, like most Jews, she had left Germany before the war started. As it happened, she, her first husband, and their three children did not get out quickly enough and were ultimately (by way of an ill-advised escape to Poland) sent to Auschwitz. She never saw her husband again after their arrival there, and the three children—four, three, and two years old—were immediately taken from her and, as she was later told, thrown into a furnace without benefit of prior treatment in the gas chamber. She had met Herman, who was Polish, in a displaced persons' camp just after the end of the war. He had never been married, but his parents and six brothers and sisters had all been killed, so he was completely alone in the world. Their wedding took place in the camp, and they had Howard quite a few years after their arrival in the United States.

Although I have heard this story, with very few variations, on many occasions, I will never get used to it. It does not matter if even the Holocaust has become a sort of industry, with commissions, museums, and television re-creations feeding off it. The very thought of children being thrown into furnaces alive, for instance, must always touch within us a raw, virgin spot that reacts to the horror of it with a passion undiminished by familiarity. For the moment, the hours and days we were spending investigating and treating every little aspect of Howard's condition seemed insanely out of proportion to the mere minutes it must have taken, door to door, to destroy her first three children. I told her so, even though it was my function to keep alive what was obviously her last and only child, and not to dig even deeper into memories that must have been much vaster and more lurid than anything her eyes ever saw in her current, everyday life.

We were still waiting for the surgeon, and for once I did not go into my usual flurry of phone calls to move things along more quickly. There was something puzzling me, and I needed an answer right away, since I am very impatient by nature. The calm and cooperative behavior of the Kalbs had not changed, even though my patient's condition had been worsening steadily since admission. As a matter of fact, and especially because I was given so much freedom of action by the family, something that made me feel even more responsible for Howard's welfare, this case agitated me no end. It was a real contradiction: the family seemed more tranquil than the doctor! I finally asked Jenny the question that had been on my mind all along. I had just said, "How can you—" when she interrupted me and said, "I know what you are going to say, Doctor, so let me make it easy for you! You were going to ask how we can look so *ruhig*"—she slipped into her native tongue for a moment, using the German word for "calm"—"when we have so much to lose. I have friends who were also in the camps, and they are nervous wrecks all the time. When anybody in their family just has a cold, they act like it's a calamity, and if they have something really bad, don't even ask how they behave!" She is right, I thought, the concentration camp survivors I have taken care of have almost always been suspicious and anxious (understandably, to say the least), and that is why I never thought that she or Herman fit in with that group. "But why," she continued, "Herman and I don't act like that is another story. You see, when we met in the DP camp, we had already lost everything we had ever had: children, husband, parents, brothers, sisters, home, everything! It was just as if we had both died and been born again, as grown-ups, in that DP camp, with our past *ausgewischt* [wiped away] and our future, of course, not written yet." She had always expressed herself very simply, yet she was eloquent now, and it was a surprise. But then again, I thought, just one more unexpected development in the Kalb saga. "In Auschwitz, a lot of people lost their religion, you can imagine why," she continued. "I never did, and continued to say my prayers every day, just like at home. But when we got out of Auschwitz, everything had already happened to Herman and me that only happens to most people in their most terrible nightmares. Don't you see, *nothing* worse than that could ever happen to us again. It's not as if we arranged it between us, but I guess we both waited to see what the future would bring. I never stopped praying, I certainly do now, all the time, for Howard to get better. But I've also known since Auschwitz that whether I cry or I laugh, or whether I complain or I accept doesn't make the slightest bit of difference. You *have* to trust somebody who is of this world. For all I know, you may be God's instrument, so how can I make you crazy and take you away, even a little bit, from taking care of my Howard?"

Unfortunately, I never had a chance to answer her provocative words because, at that very moment, damn it, the surgeon appeared. He could have waited another five minutes and given me a chance to go into her unusual thinking a little bit more! He seemed to be in a hurry, so I went right in with him and held Howard's hand while he had his tracheostomy done under local anesthesia in his cubicle in the ICU.

Even though the time never seemed right to take up the conversation with Jenny again, I realized I had gotten an insight into something very rare—namely, why people behave in a certain way, a subject that in most instances is a closed book. Happily, Howard's illness was kind enough to relent on its own (which helped to confirm Guillain-Barré as the diagnosis), and his muscle function began to improve a few days later. Soon after that, he was well enough to be discharged from the hospital. He got married recently and sent me a wedding picture. He is standing there with his bride, looking pretty much the same as the first time I ever saw him, except that now, of course, his eyelids are no longer droopy. In the background is his female counterpart, Jenny, smiling as always. She was right to trust to the future. It has done well by her!

Fortunately, I have met up with any number of families like the Kalbs, who gave me the support I needed to do what I could for their sick relatives. There were children who helped me with their parents, parents who helped me with their children, brothers and sisters and nephews and nieces who smoothed the way for me. It is remarkable how similar my experiences were with them, although the people involved and the patients' illnesses were so different. Jenny Kalb's story is, of course, unique, and I will never forget it. Yet the best way I can express my feelings about the many others who were helpful and humane is to say that I no longer remember the details of what they did or how they did it. All their kindnesses together add up to one large, warm memory that I cherish.

I remember the difficult families much better, maybe because there was such a great variety of ways in which they could be difficult. To make matters even more complicated, some relatives appeared difficult but turned out to be perfectly justified in putting roadblocks in the path of the doctors. It was not just irrational anxiety on their part but good judgment (which does not belong to doctors only) that made them question decisions about tests, medications, surgery, and so on. Experienced physicians have learned that it pays to use the knowledge that relatives carry around in the backs of their heads. A patient's old aunt may remember that he had an allergic reaction to penicillin as a child, for instance, and that may help to prevent a massive reaction now. Another patient's husband is alert enough to tell the doctor that she always bled a lot after having a tooth pulled. This is sometimes a sign of a clotting problem, and it is definitely something to investigate before she has her surgery.

Yet what if the aunt stirs up an outcry in the family against treatment with penicillin without giving the whole story? Then the doctor is left in the dark, because the only thing he hears is "We don't want him to get antibiotics; they're dangerous." Or the husband of the lady who needs surgery may keep on trying to put it off because he is afraid that she is going to bleed to death and he does not know that clotting problems can be treated. In other words, relatives may have the best intentions but can end up looking "difficult." In the long run, though, these things often become clearer, but sometimes it takes nearly as much effort to find out what the family is up to as it takes to make a diagnosis in the first place.

I first learned about family interference of another kind more than thirty years ago, during the first year of my practice. My mother had referred one of her neighbors to me, a lady in her sixties whose name was Emma Thompson. She told me that she had come "just for a checkup," but it became clear to me that something else was going on, since she could remember almost nothing of her medical history. Her husband, a tall, affable, blond-haired and blue-eyed man, had to answer most of my questions about her past, but at the same time, he did not appear to think that this was in any way unusual. Her physical examination showed nothing special, and her chest x-ray and electrocardiogram were completely normal. Yet during her time in the examining room, I noticed that, in addition to being forgetful, she was also confused about where she was, who I was, and so on. This was in the days before Alzheimer's disease was a household word, but my impression was that she had a loss of thinking power somehow connected to her age, a so-called senile dementia. When we got together in my consultation room after the examination, I told them that my most likely diagnosis was that she had hardening of the arteries of the brain but that further neurological tests were necessary before I could be sure. A brain tumor has to be ruled out in this kind of situation, but I kept that thought to myself. The tests, for which I suggested she be hospitalized, would give us the answer soon enough.

The patient did not respond at all, but her husband began to look angry, and he said, "They're all forgetful in Emma's family, there's not a damn thing wrong with her!" I tried to explain that this was not just garden-variety forgetfulness but something more than that when he cut me off, saying as he turned toward his wife, who was still staring straight ahead, "Thank you, Doctor, for being so thorough. But we don't think that Emma needs anything more than just a tonic to pep her up, do we, dear?" I tried again to convince him of the seriousness of her condition, but by this time he had helped her to get up, shook my hand, and led his wife out to the waiting room.

I was twenty-nine years old, and he was my father's age. I looked very young then (which corrected itself very quickly as I continued in practice), and the first thought that came to me was that he just did not believe me, that he did not trust my judgment. I felt terrible. My father had, of course, referred some of his patients to me because he was cutting back on his own practice, but this was the first patient my mother had ever sent me. Now I would have to tell her (without revealing any medical details, of course) that not only had her neighbor's husband not wanted to follow my advice, he had pretty much walked out on me besides. My mother must have realized that my meeting with the Thompsons had not gone well, since she mentioned to me that Mr. Thompson had not been his usual friendly self when they had met in the elevator several days after their visit to my office. She did not question me any further, though, and I was too embarrassed to say anything more about it, so we let it drop.

Over the next few days, I thought a lot about what had happened. It was really far too easy to blame myself or my youthful looks for Mr. Thompson's rejection of my advice. After all, by this time I had more than four years of intensive patient care under my belt, and I was usually able to put my point across with patients and their families, regardless of my age or appearance. I began to understand that the problem was that Mr. Thompson *believed* me, not that he didn't! He must have been angry at first because I seemed to know what was wrong with his wife, something he did not want to know. The final handshake was supposed to mean "no hard feelings," I guessed, and the quick exit from my office probably meant escape before I got any more bright ideas, rather than lack of courtesy toward me.

Denial is often used by patients and relatives when the truth of a diagnosis or the prospect of a bad outcome is too painful to face. Deep down, Mr. Thompson must have realized that his wife needed more than a tonic to get better. Yet he could not accept her drifting away from him as a social and thinking being, so he did the next best thing. He nipped my investigation in the bud, and in doing that, he came right between my patient and me. I am sure that he did not mean to harm his wife, but his attitude kept me from even trying to find a condition that I could possibly do something about.

My mother gave me the long-term follow-up, as we say.

Mrs. Thompson began to wander out of their apartment when her husband was not home, and he had to retrieve her from the local police station several times. They finally left New York and went back to their native Minnesota, and there he put her in a nursing home, where she ultimately died. On looking back, I realize she probably did have Alzheimer's, and even though there is now some experimental treatment for the disease, there was none at all at that time.

I do not know how much of a difference my making the diagnosis would have made in the long run, but she and her husband could certainly have been spared her pathetic wandering of the streets in her housecoat and her stays in the police station. If he had let me go ahead and make a diagnosis, at least I could have given him some good advice, much earlier, on how to take care of her.

Relatives can be destructive, and sometimes they use the patient's illness as a pretext for fighting psychological battles of their own. They may feel guilty because they have neglected the patient in the past, they may really dislike him but feel obligated to "care" because he is so sick, they may be in competition with other family members for the patient's affection (or, perish the thought, his inheritance), and so on. This is already the stuff of drama, but that is not surprising, because every illness, and especially one that unfolds in a hospital, is a little piece of theater all its own. Each relative has his role, one that is usually not so different from the one he or she plays in other family productions. So we have an aggressive relative, an over-solicitous one, a habitual victim, and other standard personality types. We physicians meet up with them when we play our own roles in these dramas, ranging from villain to hero (temporary, usually) to remote scientist, just to mention some of the stereotypes with which we are labeled.

There is no question, though, that relatives can throw a monkey wrench into the orderly process of patient care that the doctor has planned. Most of the time, they do not understand how complicated disease can be (and why should they? It is not their life's work), nor are they aware of the limits of the roles played by the various physicians on the case. Still, under the cover of "my relative deserves *only the best*," they feel free to manipulate one doctor against another, to hire and fire consultants, and generally to act the bull in the deceptively casual china shop where we doctors store not only our knowledge but also our determination to do as well by the patient as we humanly can.

Margie Schneider, a chunky lady in her seventies, had been a patient of mine for many years. Her husband, George, had also been under my care until he died of a heart attack when he was in his early sixties. She was very warm and funny, which endeared her to all of us in the office, but in addition she had a unique trait. Every time she came in for her appointment, she brought a dozen of the best cheese Danish any of us had ever tasted. They were individually wrapped in tissue paper, and she carried them in a plain paper box with no label. She was very vague about where these marvels originated, so their mysterious origin assumed a life of its own over the years. Ultimately, the majority opinion of the staff was that she made them herself, but that for reasons of modesty she did not want to admit that she was the genius behind the Danish.

Margie was a diabetic who did not need to take insulin. Yet she took several medications for the control of her blood pressure and for the chest pain that I thought was due to narrowing of one or more of her coronary arteries. All in all, she was, to use one of our favorite expressions, "clinically stable." This meant that her blood sugar was not too high, her blood pressure measured within acceptable limits, and, as usual, she had chest pain that came on only after a heavy meal or after walking quickly and that went away almost immediately after she put a nitroglycerin tablet under her tongue.

Her excess weight, her diabetes, and the fact that her chest pain had not changed over the years all pushed me away from doing an angiogram to see whether she needed coronary artery surgery. "If it ain't broke, don't fix it" is a saying that should have a special meaning for all doctors, and especially nowadays, when technology is often in search of subjects rather than the other way around. With Margie, I felt that things were not "broke" enough to justify doing a procedure, the angiogram, that might lead to another one, a coronary bypass, both of them with risks attached, only to end up, after a lot of suffering, with no improvement in her quality of life. Besides, it is all very well to to talk about "low" mortality or complication rates, but for the patient who is one of the unlucky 1 or 2 percent, or whatever the number is in any particular procedure, it's 100 percent!

Early one morning, at about three o'clock, my answering service woke me to tell me that Margie had called and asked me to get in touch with her right away, although she would not say what it was about. In all the years she had been my patient, Margie had never called outside of office hours, so this extraordinary call in the middle of the night could only mean that something serious was going on with her.

During all the time I was in practice, and except for vacations and some weekends when I was off call, one of the last thoughts I had before falling asleep was the possibility that I might be awakened because of some emergency. Then I would go over the prime candidates on my mental checklist—in other words, those of my patients on the outside who were worrying me, or those in the hospital whose condition was liable to change for the worse at any moment. Yet being prepared for the *possibility* of a call did not make me any less anxious when it actually happened. The ringing of the telephone, like a signal to a computer, would immediately bring the checklist to my consciousness a few moments before I became completely awake. So, with almost no delay and even in my half sleep, the suspense began. Who was in trouble? Was it one of the "official" ones from the list, the ones I had counted, as does an insomniac his proverbial sheep, while I dropped off? Or was it a "wild card," somebody completely unexpected, who had become acutely ill during the night? And not only did I think of *who* it might be, I also thought about *what if* something or other had happened to this or that one, and why I hadn't handled matters differently so as to avoid this mythical "what if." Impatience to know who it was who had called tangled with my fear of having made a wrong decision that had now come back to haunt me as I carried my cordless telephone out of the bedroom so as not to disturb my wife. I then proceeded into the bathroom, where I installed myself on my customary chair, the lid of the toilet.

Strangely enough, I was called very infrequently at night about the patients who worried me most. It should not have been that surprising, though, since I had hundreds of active patients spread out over New York City and its suburbs. So the possibility was not all that remote that, occasionally, one of them could not wait until morning to speak to me about the sudden worsening of an old condition or the worrisome beginning of a new one. Anyone who has ever been sick during the night knows that frightening feeling of being the only one in the world who is awake while everyone else in the world, it seems, is sleeping peacefully. The morning, when life comes back to its more predictable self, seems very far away, and the strong temptation is there to speak to the doctor, to be reassured by him, and to have him hold your hand, even if it is over the telephone. In my experience, most patients are very disciplined and call only when something truly alarming is going on with them, and even then they apologize sincerely. Over the years, I have rarely seen out-and-out abuse of the right every patient has to speak to his doctor (or a substitute), even at night, if the occasion demands it. Of course, the doctor is often at his worst under these circumstances. He has had a hard day, his sleep is interrupted (for good, for many of us), and he finds himself at a disadvantage in having to make decisions on the spur of the moment, without even being able to consult the patient's chart. Yet the very fact that the patient has called means, most of the time, that something serious is going on. Yet, whatever the time or the circumstances, a firm decision has to be made about what to do with the patient. "Take two aspirins and call me in the morning" is a myth. What's worse, it turns into a rumor that is spread from patient to patient. It minimizes the seriousness of the problem most patients have when they feel forced to call the doctor at night. Not only that, but it gives a false impression of the high level of concern that any experienced and conscientious doctor has for what are often the sickest patients at any one time in his practice.

As I sat in my bathroom, reminded once again that the effect of cold tile on bare feet can abruptly awaken even the sleepiest doctor, I hoped that Margie's telephone would not be busy. I have had many frustrations in medicine (after all, it is known for its many maddening moments), but there is none worse than returning the call of a patient who has phoned urgently and getting a constant busy signal. Almost always, the patient (or spouse) is speaking to a relative or is calling the doctor's office again (and likely being kept on hold by the answering service), but the possibility always exists that the patient has passed out, or died, and that the phone is off the hook for that reason. How the doctor is supposed to get through when the telephone is being used on the other end has never been clear to me, but of course the anxiety of the moment does not always make for clear thinking on the part of the patient or his family.

I was very relieved when Margie answered immediately. In this kind of situation, you take nothing for granted, and this meant that she was alive at least! She sounded a little bit more serious than usual, but still took her time in telling me her story. It seemed that she had awakened with chest pain worse than she had ever had but still in the usual location. One nitroglycerin under the tongue had always taken care of her chest pain, but she had had to take about five in the past hour, and by now the bad pain had gone away, although she still had some soreness in her chest. I asked her whether she was dizzy or sweating, and she replied that she was not, which meant to me that her blood pressure was probably not unduly low. That the chest pain had pretty much gone away with the nitroglycerin suggested that a coronary artery had not been completely closed off, but certainly the unusual timing and severity of the pain had to mean that the vessel had suddenly become much narrower.

I knew that she lived alone in the house in Nassau County, just over the New York City line, that she had shared with her husband for many years. I asked her to call the volunteer ambulance maintained by the community, and otherwise to stay off the line so I could call the paramedics back. I was very concerned. If she had had a heart attack, she belonged in the nearest coronary care unit. Yet, I knew her best and she had been a patient in my hospital before. When the paramedic later told me that she had a good blood pressure and no abnormality of her heart rhythm, and that the computerized electrocardiogram showed no evidence of a heart attack, and what's more, that the nearest hospital would take almost as much time to reach as my hospital in Manhattan, I made the decision to bring her in to New York.

It had taken about an hour to make the arrangements, and it was now about four-thirty. Going back to sleep was out of the question, especially since I wanted to see her as soon as possible. By the time she arrived in the emergency room, I was already there. Her chest pain had gone, she was her usual cheerful self, and I went about making the arrangements usual in this kind of situation. That is, I ordered tests necessary to rule in or rule out a true heart attack (meaning actual death of heart muscle), rearranged and added to her medications, tried to obtain a bed in the coronary care unit and contacted a cardiologist (the one who was taking care of my own father, by the way) for consultation.

By now it was seven A.M. I went up to the cafeteria to have breakfast, feeling that not at all unpleasant, slightly nervous rush reminiscent of the mornings after those eventful sleepless nights during my training. At this time of day, only surgeons and their residents—the latter, as always, reminiscent of warlike yet oppressed-looking marines in boot camp—were available for conversation. I decided to eat alone, and it was lucky that I did, because within fifteen minutes I began to receive repeated overhead pages. I had never met Margie's children, even during her husband's last illness. I knew that her son lived in California and her daughter in Chicago, and Margie used to complain to me, though with a smile, that "for my family, the planes only fly west," suggesting that she visited them but they did not visit her, at least not often.

It was uncanny. The messages, transmitted through my answering service, from Chicago and Los Angeles were virtually identical. The word *emergency* was used about five times in each one, and Los Angeles was "upset" and Chicago "disappointed" that Margie's neighbor had had to give them the news of her hospitalization instead of my calling them "right away." Telephone numbers were left in each case, and (after finishing breakfast, I confess) I called her children. The conversations were pretty much the same. I explained that I had been very busy during the night taking care of the practical details of getting their mother to the hospital and that I had intended to speak to Margie a little later in the morning about how and when to notify her children. My explanation was greeted with silence by Los Angeles and a curt "Sure!" by Chicago. At this point, I had to go into great detail with each one about the qualifications of my consulting cardiologist and what medicines I was giving their mother and why. Chicago was due to arrive in several hours, and I arranged to meet her during my late-afternoon rounds. Los Angeles was to arrive in the hospital at around nine P.M., and he did not ask whether he could meet me at that time but, rather, where. After I explained that I was usually at home at that hour but that I would be glad to speak to him on the telephone when he arrived at the hospital, I got another silence, which by this time I realized represented displeasure.

Margie did well. She got a bed in the coronary care unit that same day (a miracle), and she had no further chest pain. Over the next day, I met with her children. They both again grilled me (the daughter was a lawyer and the son a businessman, but he was very good at grilling also) about the cardiologist I had called in. I explained to them that I thought well enough of him to have him take care of my father, but this did not seem to impress them. They had been given the name of a particular cardiologist on our staff and they wanted him called to see their mother. I explained that he was an expert in cardiac catheterization and angiography and that I would ask him to do those procedures on Margie if she turned out to need them. I told them, however, that an experienced general cardiologist would be much more appropriate as an additional consultant. We finally agreed on a second opinion by a veteran cardiologist with superb judgment, and for the moment, an uneasy peace was maintained between them and me.

By the third day of her hospitalization, Margie was transferred to a private room. Visiting her there was, it seemed to me, probably similar to being invited to her home. Coffee (decaffeinated, in deference to her cardiac situation, I guessed) was always brewing; several dainty cups, saucers, and spoons were neatly arranged on a towel turned into a tablecloth; and those cheese Danish (my staff had been wrong, of course; their appearance at this time suggested a source other than her own kitchen) sat there plumply and invitingly. There were flowers around the room, there were open jars of candy, and in the middle of all this, Margie, in her own nightgown and bed jacket, held court. After questioning her about the past night and examining her, I would sit down to chat. I would refuse the coffee and Danish (weight gain by the doctor is one of the health hazards of hospital rounds), but I usually accepted a hard candy, and it became an instant tradition for me to put one of her flowers in my lapel.

I don't remember exactly when I first felt the chill in the air, but it must have been at some time around the end of the first week of her hospitalization. In the meantime, the condition of the relationship between her children and me was, as they say in health bulletins, "guarded." I certainly did not like them; our original telephone conversations had left a bad taste in my mouth. What's more, their requests for information always sounded like demands to me, and there was invariably a suggestion in the air that I was withholding some vital fact from them. In addition, their behavior toward me was slightly condescending, so that I always had the feeling when I spoke to them that they wondered why their mother had chosen me, of all people, to be her doctor.

What really brought about the crisis between us, though, was the call I received one morning. It was my custom not to interrupt one patient's visit by speaking on the phone to another one. Patients and relatives were on their honor, though, so if they said it was an emergency they were put through to me, no questions asked. Although people occasionally took advantage of the system, claiming that it was an emergency when they just did not want to have to wait for a call later on, the arrangement worked. It was the only way, because no matter how well my secretary knew our patients, the decision about what is an emergency is strictly a medical one, and so only one person could make it, and that was me.

Margie's daughter was on the phone. I was surprised to learn she had something "very urgent" to report to me, since I had seen her mother, who had appeared fine, within the hour. It seemed that Margie had heartburn and that "the family"—in other words, she and her brother—wanted a second opinion from a gastroenterologist! I told her that since I had not even known of the heartburn until that moment, there was not even a first opinion as yet, so a second opinion seemed premature. I then tried to reassure her that the heartburn very likely came from the many medications she was taking for her heart and that I would prescribe something as soon as I had a chance to go back to see her, which would be that afternoon. She agreed, though very reluctantly, and I sensed that this was not the end of the story. I was right, because ten minutes later her brother was on the line. He was not satisfied with either my explanation or my plan, and when, in my exasperation, I told him the first thing that came into my mind, that consulting a gastroenterologist at the first sign of heartburn is like calling in the National Guard because of a candy store break-in, he insisted that I do what he asked or he would go to the hospital administration and force me to do it.

I have always felt that one of the most important functions of a doctor is to guide his patients and their families through the confusion that surrounds sickness. In medicine, as in many other fields, things are rarely what they seem. In this case, for instance, Margie's heartburn might have frightened her children, but it was really not serious, and, as a matter of fact, it was to be expected. A family, because of its fear for the patient's well-being, may understandably jump the gun sometimes in asking that a consultant be called. Normally, though, the relatives will go along with the doctor if he can give them some good reasons why the request is premature. With this particular family, there was no persuading and no guiding, and I did not doubt that they would do as they threatened if I did not put into effect their ridiculous notion of a heartburn (I could not dignify it as a gastrointestinal) consultation. Since hospital administrators are notorious for their waffling, and since they invariably protect the hospital rather than the doctor, I had no great hope of having them in my corner if the children did complain about me. It is true that I could have agreed to their demands right away, but I chose to resist because I have always believed that a doctor, in order to have the courage to take care of patients, must also have the courage of his convictions. In this case, though, I knew I was beaten, so I called a gastroenterologist who was not only very capable but who also had a good sense of humor. I knew that he would understand.

How can you tell if a patient's feelings have changed toward you? My father has always told me to watch out when they stop smiling at you, that that is the first indication of a change of heart. In Margie's case, I first felt it as I walked into her room one day. It was just a suggestion of coldness, the kind you feel when you stand close to a frosty window in an otherwise warm room; yet it was unmistakable. She did *not* give me her usual smile of greeting that morning, and if I needed any more indication that something was seriously wrong I had only to look at the usually open, but now tightly shut, boxes of candy around the room, as well as at the now unreachable vases from which, in comparison to the days before, plucking a flower for my lapel now would have been a gross exercise. I knew what had happened. Her children had obviously spoken to her about their relationship with me. I had no idea of what they had said, but it was clear that despite our long relationship she had chosen to go along with their version of what had happened. In the previous days, I had stayed away from talking to her about my problems with her children. Although she was better, her condition was still serious enough that it could only be harmful for her to be in the middle of a struggle between her children and her doctor. By this time I was very resentful, because she had abruptly changed her attitude toward me without even trying to find out my side of the story. Yet I knew better than to get into a controversy with her. Certainly my feelings were hurt, especially because I felt that her children had victimized me from the start although I had always taken good care of her. Still, one twinge of chest pain felt by a sick lady like this in response to an emotional discussion with her doctor is much more significant than all the hurt feelings in the world, and that has to be avoided, however unfair it all is.

I never heard from her children again, and I noted that they had adopted one of the cardiologists on the case as the new official spokesman. She finally had her angiogram, which did *not* suggest that a bypass was necessary, and after that we decided to discharge her from the hospital. On the day she was to go home, I went to see her in order to give her her prescriptions, to order outpatient blood tests, to give her diet directions, and so on. But I was like the proverbial husband; I was the last to know. She told me that arrangements had already been made for her to be seen by another doctor on the outside and that my services were no longer necessary.

I had never really considered the likelihood that Margie would fire me, despite all the warning signs that should have made it quite obvious to me. Looking back on it, I find it amazing that I could have been so blind, especially considering her children's hostility and Margie's growing unfriendliness. My denial was powerful, and I think that it was because of the intense emotion and effort that I had poured into this case. There was anger at her children for coming between my good old patient, Margie, and me. There was anger at Margie for allowing her children to turn her away from her good old doctor. There was a feeling of being unappreciated for my conscientious care, especially during the first night and in the emergency room. And there was also another very human emotion involved: resentment at being discarded, at being passed over unjustly in favor of the cardiologist I had personally selected.

Like any other doctor, especially a busy one, I have had my share of patients who have left me in order to go to someone else. As they say, it comes with the territory, and it is something that cannot be avoided. Yet every time I received a release for a patient's records to be sent somewhere else, I felt vaguely unhappy for a while. The temptation was always there for me to think that it was all my fault that the patient was leaving, that it was something I did that had prompted the break. Realistically, of course, there are many reasons other than personality differences or disenchantment with the doctor's management of a case that lead to a patient's decision to leave. Yet it is one thing to receive a written release and to sulk about it in the privacy of your office, and it is quite another to be fired by a patient personally. I was very embarrassed. I did not know what to say at first, or whether to stand up or sit down; my face suddenly felt hot, yet I hoped I didn't look as if I were blushing, and so on. I finally just wished her well, shook her hand, and walked out.

A few months ago, I heard through one of my other patients that Margie had died. I still think about what happened between us now and then, and I know that it will always make me a little sad.

6

Bad News

URING MEDICAL SCHOOL and the training period afterward, we are all exposed to some very unpleasant sights, smells, and experiences. A gangrenous foot, for example, is very ugly, and the smell of its decomposing flesh can never be forgotten after the first time it hits the novice's up to now innocent nostrils. Death, whether it is first encountered in the formaldehyde-soaked anatomy class cadaver or later, when it has just transformed the live patient of a minute before into his identical twin who is sleeping some incomprehensible sleep, is never an event to be taken casually. Yet habit and our lessening squeamishness (we hope) combine to take the edge off the horror on the daily menu. We certainly do not become indifferent, but we realize, even early on, that we have to get beyond these inevitable assaults on our senses if we are to do anything more than gag and run out of the room each time we encounter them.

Yet there is one part of being a doctor I have never been able to get used to and that I have always considered to be an emotional burden: that is, to be the bearer of bad news. Don't mistake my calm look, my smile, the relaxed way in which I sit behind my desk or on the edge of the bed as I tell you about the biopsy that shows cancer or as I advise you to have major heart surgery. I am a professional, and my first obligation is to you. I cannot cry with you, because you depend upon me to be

104

strong and to maintain emotional control. But I *feel* along with you just the same, and since I have had to be the messenger for literally thousands of unhappy communiqués in my medical lifetime, it should come as no great surprise to me that, each time I explode this ominous little bomb, that sensitive old spot within me hurts all over again.

However traumatic it is for him personally, the doctor is the only one who can convey critical information to the patient and his family. It is not in his power to reverse bad news, but it is definitely within his province to soften the blow, while at the same time not tampering too much with the truth. We doctors often make the mistake of thinking that our patients have a lot more knowledge than they actually do. Most patients do not even know what questions to ask in order to measure for themselves the significance of this or that "bad diagnosis." What to tell a patient, and how, requires a game plan. The patient's personality and what the doctor knows about his emotions have to be taken into account. Since these are unique, the way in which bad news is presented has to be carefully tailored to the individual patient as well.

For years now, I have tried very hard to keep other doctors from giving diagnoses, especially serious ones, to my patients on an impromptu, unprepared basis. I have had some very disagreeable experiences where, for instance, the resident on six A.M. rounds, and while the patient is still in a half sleep, casually says to his team, "It's colon cancer, all right. We'll have to take it out," as he leaves the room without another word. The patient is, of course, terrified and does not even know whether he heard correctly. Afterward, when the damage has already been done, it is very difficult to go back and start all over again in the right way. And yet, the future of the patient—how well he accepts an operation or chemotherapy, let's say—depends on how well and how humanely the whole process is explained to him in the first place.

The doctors who blurt out diagnoses are probably as uncomfortable with giving bad news as I am. But they want to get rid of the information as quickly as possible—in other words, to shift the burden from themselves to the patient, and in the process they cause great distress all around.

But then again, is it really necessary to tell the patient everything? Complete honesty on the part of the doctor *sounds* wonderful and confidence-inspiring, but it can sometimes make the patient worse. Certainly I have met up with any number of strong characters who want to be told *whatever* is wrong with them and who don't lose their composure after I give them bad news. But there are others, quite a few, as a matter of fact, who have to be handled much more carefully. They are the ones who send mixed signals, because in addition to saying, "I can take it, tell me what's wrong, whatever it is," they ask in the same breath, "I don't have cancer, do I?" Experienced physicians know that the question is really a plea and that the patient does not want nearly as much information as he would like it to appear.

Of course, patients have to be told what is going on if they require an operation, for example. You cannot recommend removal of part of the colon and yet not tell the patient that he has colon cancer. But if, later on, the tumor has spread, it is not necessary to go over the whole list of organs that are affected. This excessive frankness can only make him even more discouraged and less willing to help himself by continuing his fight against the disease. In this kind of situation, it is enough to talk of "some" spread and to hold out the hope that further treatment can take care of it. I am not suggesting that we lie to patients or that we give them empty reassurances. What I am suggesting, though, is that doctors fulfill their function as interpreters for their patients. It takes courage and the willingness to take responsibility to do this, as well as the ability to keep things to themselves if necessary. In this case at least, shutting up can be a virtue and unnecessary honesty a crime.

Olga Kessler became my patient in the mid-1960s and was at that time about fifty-five. When I first saw her, it seemed to me that she was easily one of the most fearful patients I had ever seen, and even now, many years later, she is still high up on the list. She'd had a kidney cancer removed about ten years before, and she focused all her anxiety on spread of the tumor. Her previous doctor had retired, and from what I could see in the chart she brought with her, as well as from my examination, she seemed to be well. Yet she cried off and on when we first met, and she admitted that she spent many hours of the day, as well as a great part of her sleepless nights, worrying about what would happen when (never if) her tumor "comes back." Her husband was with her and murmured little words of reassurance to her, to which she responded occasionally with a little smile and a squeeze of his hand. His part in this obviously well rehearsed ritual had only a temporary effect, though, because she immediately began to sigh and weep all over again as soon as she let go of his hand. His hands did not stay at rest, though, and I noticed that they were shaking. He did not have the appearance of someone with Parkinson's disease, so I thought I was being clever by tying his trembling to the nervousness I thought his wife's constant complaining must have produced in him. But it turned out that he was a sculptor, and the trembling came from fifty years of chiseling and hammering stone. So much for fancy, premature clinical conclusions!

Olga had a mixture of severe anxiety and depression. She had been seen by psychiatrists over the years, but she had not been able to stand various combinations of tranquilizers and antidepressants, which had made her either more depressed or more anxious. I realized that reassurance would have a very temporary effect on driving away her fears and that she would require a lot of emotional support instead. This term is, of course, very vague, and means different things to different doctors. As far as I am concerned, though, it cannot be prescribed like a medicine or thought of as a quick fix, like surgery. The doctor has to give something of himself in this situation, something he cannot take back and that acts like a foundation for whatever little bit of courage and optimism the patient can still produce.

Right from the beginning, I told Olga that I did not expect to be able to take away her fears about the cancer but that I would do my very best to watch for it and to hit it as hard and as quickly as I could if it did come back. In the meantime, I asked her to call as often as she needed to, or to come to the office even without an appointment when she felt she could no longer cope with her feelings of terror. I don't pretend that a dramatic improvement took place after our first meeting, but the fact that I was available to her, and did not try to talk her out of anything, must have helped a little bit. At first, she telephoned frequently and showed up unannounced a few times. Later on, we saw each other only on scheduled visits, and I took that as an encouraging sign of at least some improvement in her condition.

About a year after her first visit, Olga came in one day complaining of "pain all over." She was crying and groaning very much as she had at the beginning, and she assured me that this time the cancer *had* come back. Kidney cancer is notorious for its spread to bone, but I kept that to myself. I did tell her that she needed to be examined and that some tests had to be done, but for all we knew she might just have a bad case of arthritis. As it happened, she turned out to have multiple myeloma, a form of bone cancer that had nothing to do with her original kidney tumor. The blood tests and x-rays were typical for the diagnosis, and as far as I was concerned, that is what she had. The only thing left to be done was a bone marrow examination, and that would be necessary only if we were going to start treatment.

I had some very difficult choices to make. Not only did Olga have cancerophobia (an exaggerated fear of cancer), she also had cancer. There was really only one treatment for myeloma at the time, but the medication was frequently ineffective. On the one hand, the myeloma was sure to kill her if she was not treated. On the other hand, especially because she was so suspicious, we could not do a bone marrow and then give her (what was at that time primitive) chemotherapy without informing her of what we were doing. Yet if we told her that she had cancer, it was very possible that she would go into an even deeper depression, one that might even require shock therapy. Yet shock therapy could cause fractures in bones riddled with myeloma, and so on, and so on.

I add all these "on the other hands" and "yets" to my thoughts to show the impossible situation we were in. What's more, there was no strict right or wrong to point us in the proper direction. I finally came to the conclusion that the only thing we could hope for in this frustrating case was damage control, and nothing more.

I spent a lot of time thinking about what to do, and I conferred with several older internists and also with a psychiatrist whose common sense I respected. Yet I knew that in the long run it was going to have to be my call—after a discussion with the family, of course. Since the medication often did not help, there was a real case to be made for telling her that she had arthritis, treating her with painkillers, and letting her die without having to face the knowledge that she had cancer, the illness that terrified her most. But what if she belonged to the small group of people who had a dramatic response to the medication? Was it fair to let her die without even giving her the chance to live?

I called in her husband and her daughter as soon as I had

the reports, and I presented the problem to them. When I told them the news, her husband's hands shook more than ever, so I guessed that I had been a little right, after all. He had, of course, witnessed her terrible fear for over ten years, and at first he begged me not to tell her the truth. Her daughter, on the other hand, wanted her mother to have every chance to live, whatever the odds. We talked back and forth for several hours, and I admit that I wavered a lot, sometimes siding with one, sometimes with the other, which just demonstrated my own conflict. Finally, we exhausted all the arguments and came to a decision. Since my particular variety of emotional support had seemed to work with Olga before, I would tell her what she had, though putting it in the mildest possible terms, and we would all be very positive and optimistic about the treatment. Telling her had won out very narrowly over not telling her, and I must say that I had a lot of misgivings over whether we were doing the right thing.

She came to my office the next day, and I did what parents learn how to do: give bitter medicine with a cube of sugar. She took the news surprisingly well; that is, with dry eyes and a calm look. I told her that I had made arrangements for her to be admitted to the hospital the next day, and when she left, she said, "I'll see you." That night, after her husband had gone to sleep, she jumped out the window.

Olga was the exception and not the rule. Most anxious patients, even when they are told the very frightening truth, do not kill themselves. But giving certain patients news that they cannot tolerate can have the same effect as giving them a toxic dose of a medication; that is, even if they do not die from it, they will certainly be worse after it is administered. Of course, how much and what kind of news to give does not depend only on the doctor. Families often have very definite opinions, and these have to be taken into account. Yet what I learned from Olga's case is that I should have stuck to what I remember was my instinct at the time, and that was to let her die without confirming her worst fears rather than risking her poor, fragile emotions on the crazy wager that the chemotherapy would work. I have also realized since then that it is not the function of the doctor to accommodate or to take part in a compromise. He is not there to be a peacemaker for the family. He is there to give his best opinion, based upon his knowledge and experience. If the doctor truly believes that the patient might have a possibly shorter but still-happier life if he is not told something he cannot accept, then that is the best advice. If family or legal considerations go against the doctor's opinion, then he will at least have been an honest advocate for the protection of his patient.

Most of the time, of course, it is the doctor who is the pipeline of knowledge to the patient. He receives the raw data (laboratory numbers, x-ray reports, and the like) from the appropriate sources, throws them into the blender with his own findings, and ends up with a product that he hopes will help the patient understand, in everyday language, what is wrong with him. Patients absolutely cannot do without this middleman, not only because medicine and illness make up a foreign language that must be interpreted for them, but also because the relative significance of individual findings has to be made clear to them. Patients are constantly tempted to use their expertise in, let's say, law or architecture or plumbing or clothing manufacturing in trying to figure out some of the ins and outs of medicine, so I say this as a very well meant warning and not to show how wonderful we doctors are. Medicine is complicated and sneaky, and all too often it does not even follow its own rules! So don't go into this jungle alone, and be sure to take along a guide whom you trust.

There are times, though, when patients control the flow on their own, and in this way they may end up with either more or less information than was offered by the doctor. For example, one of the doctors in the x-ray department at the hospital once referred his parents to me for general medical care. They were in their early sixties and both had high blood pressure that needed to be followed, yet neither had any particular complaints. On their initial visit, I picked up a skin cancer on the husband and a breast mass on his wife. The cancer was removed, and the mass turned out to be benign on biopsy, so the entire family praised me highly for my thoroughness. Doctors not only need constant reassurance about how good they are, they also love to show off in front of other doctors. So in this particular case I had it all, and I was very pleased with myself. There was only one problem. Every time the patients came in for their blood pressure check, I found something new on the limited physical examination I did at those times. Once I heard a new heart murmur on the husband, which led to a cardiac echo test and a cardiology consultation. Another time, I found the wife's spleen slightly enlarged, and we were obligated to try to find the cause of that particular finding.

The patients looked more and more frightened every time they came to see me, and I could not blame them, especially since there seemed to be no end to the things I was finding on them. Finally, they had had enough. On their last visit, the husband said, "Dr. Berczeller, you are easily the most compulsive doctor we have ever seen, and that's one of the reasons our son sent us to you. But neither my wife nor I can tolerate the tension of coming here and waiting, as it happens, *every damn time* for you to find something new. We have talked it over. We can't stand it anymore! Our son is sure to be angry at us, but we're willing to take the risk of not knowing about something that might turn out to be dangerous in the long run. We know you mean well, and we're grateful for what you have done for us, but we're switching to a doctor who is not going to examine us so much all the time. We may turn out to be sicker a while from now, but in the meantime we'll be happier." I really could not blame them, and if I had been in their situation I might very well have done the same thing. They had made an emotional decision to know *less*, and as we parted warmly I assured them of my respect for them and their choice.

What about patients who want to know *more* than may be good for them? Is it reasonable to insist on having a test taken for a particular incurable illness when you have no symptoms and very negligible, if any, risk factors?

As a general internist at a major university medical center, I did not take care of AIDS patients, since the infectious disease specialists and hematologists were much more knowledgeable and experienced in this field. Yet since the initial and yearly physicals of all my patients included screening blood work, it was not unusual for someone to request that an AIDS test be included. We take it for granted that people often lie to themselves as well as to the doctor, and I cannot vouch for the fact that some of these men and women did not have some risky episodes in their past, like homosexual or bisexual contact or intravenous drug abuse. I do not think that I am being particularly naive, though, if I say that I believed the majority of them when they said, in one way or another, "I thought I'd just check, to make sure." At this point, I would go into their history again, to be absolutely certain that I had not overlooked some good reason the test should be done. But I also felt obligated to tell them that an HIV test is not harmless and that the knowledge of a positive test is sure to create great emotional suffering way before any symptoms appear. Since there is no cure for AIDS as yet, and since treatment with various drugs before any abnormal cell counts or symptoms appear is still a matter for discussion, isn't there a case to be made for *not* knowing prematurely? Certainly there are exceptions to my advice, the most important being the danger of spreading the disease. But if patients are already using condoms and not engaging in high-risk activities that can spread AIDS—in other words, if they cannot be any "better" than they already are—why look for trouble and know something devastating for what is often a long time, and yet not be able to do anything about it? Mine may not be the "correct" public health approach, and I cannot really blame those who want to identify every last HIV-positive person in the country. Yet I have always dealt with individuals and not with statistics, so I feel justified in trying to protect at least my small group from a possibly unnecessary and certainly catastrophic intrusion into their lives.

Although withholding certain frightening facts from specific patients is a time-honored strategy for maintaining their often very shaky emotional balance, I do not want to create the impression that this well-meant and well-thought-out tampering with the truth applies to the majority of our patients. On the contrary, most of the time we must tell them when we pick up something wrong on their physical examination or on their tests, especially since we need their cooperation and understanding if we are to do a decent investigation for the cause of the abnormality. "Don't worry about it, just do what I tell you" does not genuinely reassure patients nowadays and, if anything, makes them more anxious, since it gives full play to their imagination. Any even halfway busy doctor has to give unpleasant news of varying "badness" to patients and their families almost every day that he practices. Sometimes it is an already sick patient who is not better or who is even worse, and other times there is one who shows up with a worrisome new symptom or, let us say, a lump that he has found on himself. The doctor has to respond each time; he has to say *something* that makes sense and that, by the very fact that it keeps the dialogue going, leaves the impression that there is hope, that he is paying attention, and that he is doing his best. The patient and his relatives must never be made to feel that the doctor has given up. That is the cruelest blow and leaves them defenseless at the very time when they need us most.

It is really a hard choice to make, to decide which of the many unpleasant experiences having to do with the spreading of bad news is the most devastating for any particular doctor. For me, hands down, it is when I have to tell an unsuspecting, well patient who is in for a routine checkup that I have found something that may well be serious.

Ruth Herman is a fifty-two-year-old woman who is in for her annual physical. She has been my patient for fifteen years, and aside from an enlarged thyroid, she has been well throughout. She sees her gynecologist regularly for an examination and a Pap smear, and usually has her annual mammography during the week after her visit to me. When I come into the examining room, we greet each other affectionately. She is petite and energetic and still speaks with the English accent she brought here with her after her marriage to an American serviceman. She has just retired from teaching, and since I know that her son lives in California, we chat about her last visit there and about her granchildren. Today's chest x-ray is on the view box, along with last year's, and I am happy to see that the scars from her old tuberculosis have not changed in the interval. Her electrocardiogram is, as usual, normal. Her blood and urine have been collected, so I am ready to catch up on her history since our last meeting and to examine her. As I question her about her appetite, medications that she may be taking that have been prescribed by other doctors, and whether she has had any recent illnesses, I note her weight and compare it with last year's. I then take her blood pressure in both arms, make a note of it, and will tell her about it afterward. Some very anxious patients cannot wait for the details until the end of the visit, and for them I provide a "play by play," in other words, a running commentary on the results of the examination as I am performing it. But Ruth is a calm person by nature, and English to boot, so I have never felt the need to give her a moment-to-moment bulletin of my findings. I then proceed to record her pulse rate, check her reflexes, and use a tuning fork to check for the sense of vibration in her feet. Meanwhile, I am starting the so-called systemic review, in which I ask her about specific symptoms related to various organ systems. At the same time, I am examining her head, eyes (including the retina on both sides), ears, nose, and throat, as well as her thyroid, which I am glad to see has not increased in size any further. I feel around her neck for enlarged lymph nodes (there are none) and find nothing unusual during my examination of the heart and lungs. By this time I have reached the digestive system on the systemic review (having already covered headaches, vision, hearing, the upper and lower respiratory tracts, and the heart), and so far there are no disquieting symptoms.

I always examine the breasts with the patient both sitting *and* lying down, and I remind her of this before I start so she will not think, when I do the repeat examination, that I have found something wrong on the first one. First I look at the breasts and the nipples, and I see no suspicious bumps. I feel the right breast going from one sector to the next and repeat the examination with her right arm raised and her right hand behind her head. I am satisfied, and I say to her, "Number one okay!" We both laugh. "Boy, do I hate this part of it," she says, and I think to myself, You and me both, kid!

When we want to identify an abnormal finding in the breast, we have to have an address for it so we can revisit it when the time has come to decide what to do about it. For this reason, the breast is divided like a map into sections, in this case called quadrants (in other words, quarters of this half-grapefruit-shaped organ tacked on to the chest wall). So my fingers walk from the upper outer to the lower outer and upper inner to lower inner quadrants, and at regular intervals plumb deeper in their house-to-house search for any fugitive mass that might be hiding there.

These fingers are in a very delicate situation, though, because they belong to people who on the one hand are searching for lumps but who on the other hand are fervently hoping that there are none there. This conflict comes to the surface especially when the message is sent by one of these extensions of ourselves that they have hit pay dirt, that they have done what they are supposed to do, in other words, that they have found something. Yet, instead of praise for a job well done, the return message is often one of disbelief together with the order to check again, and this time better news, please! And this is what turned out to happen with Ruth. While I was examining the upper outer quadrant of the left breast, I felt something the size of a cherry pit that had the consistency of a wet cotton ball—in other words, it was not as hard as a pit, yet not nearly as soft as the rest of the breast. The first impulse, when you are involved in a situation like this, is to pounce on the suspicious spot, to squeeze it and roll it and pull it, almost as if an admission of its true identity could, by some miracle, be choked out of it. But this sudden change in the otherwise flowing rhythm of the examination is frightening to the patient, who is immediately aware that something is wrong. The experienced doctor has learned not to miss a step, even when he feels or sees something abnormal, to go on as if nothing has happened, and then to sweep back for another feel or look. He also knows that the temptation to express the shock of discovery verbally, saying "Oops" or "Wait a minute" at a critical time during the examination, is insensitive and must be resisted, whatever his surprise at the unexpected finding.

The next several minutes—that is, in the time elapsed between the initial alarm sent out by my fingers and the moment when I felt it would be safe to go back again—are, as always, excruciating. I know very well that if I feel the lump again I have to believe that it is really there. If it turns out not to be a cancer, she will have had a scare that she will never forget. And if it is a cancer, this visit will turn out to be *the* turning point of her life. As in a flash, I can see the road ahead. The operation, the tests, the scans, the wait for the lymph node results (do they show spread or not?), the decision about chemotherapy, and so on, and so on, and so on.

I find myself delaying the reexamination of the suspicious area. Deep down I know that the lump is real, but on some level I must figure that, as long as I have not confirmed it, she and I are spared the truth for at least another few minutes. By now, I have asked her to lie down on her back and am going through the last few questions in the systemic review. I feel and listen to her abdomen, check the pulses in her legs and feet, again listen to her heart, finally put a finger into her rectum, and check the stool on the glove for blood. The grace period is over. There is nothing left to do but to check the breasts again, and when I do, there is no question that I was right the first time. Now there is no way out, either for her or for me. I have to tell her what I have found.

I had always given Ruth the results of my physical (the laboratory results were, of course, not yet available) while she was still in the examining room. Changing the usual procedure and asking her to meet me "for a talk" in my consultation room this time would have just created unnecessary suspense for her. So I asked her to sit on the examining table, and I settled down on my little rolling swivel stool. I took one last, farewell look at her old self, the easy way in which she sat there, the trusting, untroubled set of her face. She was probably planning the rest of her afternoon in the city, I thought, or figuring whether she would have time, after leaving my office, to catch the next bus back to her home in Rockland County. It seemed to me that at that exact moment she was no different from an unsuspecting passenger on an airliner that is going to crash and whose only concerns are about where his relatives will be picking him up or whether he will make his connecting flight on time.

I spoke of a game plan before, of the different approaches that have to be used with different patients when there is no way to avoid giving them alarming news. Ruth was a rational, unhysterical person, and I felt that it was best to play to that particular strength of hers. I knew that she would accept the news without much outward emotion, but, in my experience, "unflappability" in no way reflects the emotional upheaval this information unleashes within the patient. It is only the inexperienced doctor who takes for granted that outer and inner composure go hand in hand. It is far wiser to assume that *every* patient, whatever his exterior, needs explanation, encouragement, and gentle delving into the fearful fantasies that inevitably come along when he begins to reflect on what has happened to him.

So I told her, straight out, that she had a lump in her breast. The effect was instantaneous. First the smile went, and almost immediately after that, her face turned white. My tendency in these situations is to keep on talking, to get in as many reassuring facts as possible, to try to neutralize even a little bit the effect of the terrible thing that I have told someone. What I really try to do is to anticipate many of the patient's questions and, early in the game, give her ammunition to fight the despair she is bound to feel when the significance of what she has been told begins to sink in. I have always reassured patients on the basis of facts and not on the basis of lies. But just as any good lawyer does for his client, I use these facts to put my patient and his problems in the best possible light. I use the most benign interpretation there is for the realities that cannot be changed.

Fortunately, there were many hopeful aspects to Ruth's situation. First of all, I told her, we were not even sure what the lump really was. It might not even be a cancer, I added. But if it was, it was small and there were no enlarged lymph nodes in her armpits suggesting spread. What I did not tell her, though, was that you do not have to feel lymph nodes involved by cancer, that often the cancer is picked up only by the microscope. What's more, I told her that I was encouraged that she looked and felt so well and that I had found no other abnormalities on her examination. I did not go into statistics and I did not yet go into various combinations of treatment for breast cancer. All I did was prepare the groundwork for the likelihood that it was a malignancy, but at the same time I used all the optimistic pieces of information I could think of, to reassure not only her but myself as well.

Ruth had been completely silent up to this point and had not even tried to interrupt my monologue. She had nodded, as if in agreement, from time to time, but I had the feeling that she had not absorbed much, not surprising considering how recently I had given her the shocking news. Now, though, and she must have been more aware than I had thought, she asked me just one question: "Dr. Berczeller, what do you *really* think this lump is?" She did not use any of the stock phrases like "I can take it" and so on, but I knew (actually, I had always known) that I could be frank with her. I replied that I thought that she had cancer, esspecially because the lump had appeared during her menopause and also because she had never in the past had the cysts and benign growths in her breasts that many women have. A little bit of color had come back into her face by now, and although she still appeared a little shaky, it seemed to me that we could start talking about what to do next.

Personally, I hate uncertainty, and I am always made anxious and terribly dismayed by a reminder, such as in Ruth's case, of how unpredictable life can be and how vulnerable all we human beings are. Waiting for the other shoe to drop is something I also dread, and I am sure that it is this psychological trait of mine that was responsible for the rapid workups I performed on many of my patients. If a patient had an occasional ache in his abdomen, I did not object to his having to wait for a sound wave test of the gallbladder for a few days. But I have always considered it unacceptable, for instance, to make a woman wait for days and days for a mammogram after a breast mass has been felt on her, and then, if surgery is found to be necessary, to schedule the operation for a few weeks from then. Patients are so used to being just that, patient, that they do not adequately complain about delays that are bound to make them even more anxious than they already are. How significant is a schedule compared with the fears that patients have, in the middle of the night, about what is wrong with them and, consequently, how long they are going to live? Are the economics of the hospital or the desire of doctors for "normal" working hours more important than relieving the torture of uncertainty in these situations?

The consultants I worked with were used to my frequent calls for urgent action, so when I called Julie, an excellent and very busy mammographer, and explained the situation to her, she agreed to do the procedure right away. When Ruth came back to my office, I had already received the report by telephone, and it was, as I had suspected, a cancer of the breast. She was, understandably, subdued, but again very calm. She needed a biopsy, of course, and now it was a question of choosing the surgeon. Technically, the three or four who did most of the breast surgery at my hospital were equally competent. Yet as personalities they were very different. I canceled out two of them immediately because they were both so excitable that I sent only overtly nervous patients to them. The match of anxious surgeon with anxious patient worked out very well in these cases, but my very collected Ruth needed someone more along the lines of her own temperament. Rob, an older general surgeon who was now doing only breast procedures and who betrayed his Scots descent by his reticent and conservative manner, fit the bill very well. It was early evening by then, and I reached him at home. I explained what had happened to Ruth during her terrible afternoon and asked him to speak to her. Not only did he give her an appointment for early the next morning, he must also have given her a lot of encouragement. By the time she hung up the telephone, her face had come back to its usual pink color, and at least the charming curling up of both sides of her lips, if not her usual full smile, had come back as well.

She and Rob decided on a lumpectomy and node dissection. Happily, the lymph nodes showed no spread of the cancer and she was put on hormone therapy. When I last saw her three years after I first picked up the lump, the cancer had not shown itself again. Invariably, when we get together, the conversation always comes back to that memorable afternoon, and we talk as do veterans of a long-ago campaign. Yet, unlike old men who want to stop time, Ruth and I would like to rush it forward. We would both like her to have already reached those magical multiples of five: a five-year, a ten-year, a fifteen-year survival. When I look at her now, I can bring back the picture my memory took of her at the instant before I gave her the bad news. On the surface, nothing seems to have changed. But she knows, as I do, that she will never be the same again.

7

Playing God

WHEN A PATIENT asks, "Do you want to hear a doctor joke?" I have learned to duck because the pie is speeding toward my face as we speak. Patients often use harmless jokes as a way of breaking the ice in their dialogue with the doctor. Yet occasionally, the story with a funny ending is told for another reason, though one that may not at all be apparent to the storyteller. Just as "dirty" jokes are usually demeaning to women or to homosexuals and dialect jokes frequently have racist undertones, "doctor" jokes rarely have to do with how much people love us or respect us. But they are meant to send a message, so this is why I take these oblique exercises in humor seriously.

About fifteen or twenty years ago, a patient told me a funny little story that turned out to have a large impact on my understanding of the relations between patients and doctors. I don't remember the patient's name anymore, or what his beef was, so it appears that my memory, in some spasm of economy, chose to keep his story but discarded everything else about him.

It seems that Saint Peter is showing a visitor around heaven. While he is explaining to him that, contrary to popular belief, God's function is only that of chairman of the board and that He has no influence on anything that happens in the universe, they come upon Him sitting in front of a giant microphone. As

He barks orders such as "So-and-so has to die," "XYZ has to be pulled out at the last second," and "The flu epidemic is to stop *today*," the visitor turns to his guide and says, "I thought you told me that God doesn't have any direct executive power!" Saint Peter answers, with a finger to his lips, "Shh, not so loud! Today's His day to play doctor."

Whether a doctor *should* play God (not that he really can, of course) is a source of confusion not only for patients but for doctors as well. Patients, however sophisticated they are, must sometimes dream of having their health and lives totally influenced by a benevolent power not under their control. At the same time, the very thought of so much control in the hands of another human being may make them frightened and resentful.

Doctors are, of course, conflicted as well. On the one hand, they know the outer limits of what science and medicine can do. On the other, to be so close and yet so far from the real ability to influence the patient's fate makes them frustrated. As a result, they sometimes talk themselves into believing that they have far more influence than they actually do. This, in turn, leads to anything from unnecessary meddling in people's lives to false reassurances and baseless treatments, all of which work to the great disadvantage of the patient.

Yet there are situations where even the most rational doctor is faced with an excruciating choice. It may be, for example, that he has some special knowledge about the patient or his relative, and that the temptation is there to balance the scales, to right a wrong—in other words, to do good by using this godlike overview. Or the temptation may be there to stop a life when its owner begs to be released from his senseless suffering. And, as yet another example, how far should a doctor go if he has received privileged information that a healthy, nonpsychotic individual is about to commit suicide for reasons that are "understandable"?

*   *   *

Alton and Valerie Beale had been referred to me in the mid-1960s by my father at around the time he was retiring from his practice. Alton was a robust, handsome man in his late fifties with an intact head of close-cropped white hair, and his authoritative manner spoke for the many years he had spent as a top executive of a large international furniture company. Yet he was also very ingratiating, especially with women, as it turned out. Even on his first visit to my office, he was immediately on a first-name, kidding basis with both my secretary and my technician. Unfortunately, though, despite appearing to be well, he had high blood pressure as well as severe coronary artery disease, so he required multiple medications to control these two related problems. Despite all this, he seemed remarkably cheerful. When I questioned him about his sexual function, especially because of the known lessening of potency by some of the medications he was taking, he answered with a worldly wink and a terse "Nobody's been complaining!"

Valerie, in contrast, had no medical problems. Yet, despite the fact that this was only our first meeting, she lost no time in describing to me the depth of her unhappiness. She was Alton's fourth wife, and had had an affair with him while he was running his company's English subsidiary and was still living with his third wife. When they moved to New York, a few months before we met and very soon after his divorce and their marriage, she encountered some very unpleasant surprises.

The first was about money. He had never told her that he was paying alimony to his first two wives, only that he had to "pay off" his most recent wife so that he could marry Valerie. In addition, he had four children from his various marriages, all of them requiring his support as well. Valerie had never been married, had always worked, and, obviously unrealistically, had "looked forward to a gracious life in America with my handsome new husband." Instead, they lived, according to her, "in a dreary apartment" on lower Third Avenue, not a stylish area, and she had had to go back to work.

Not only that, but he had never told her how sick he was, how little he could do without having chest pain, and how much the medicines affected him.

"In what way do they affect him?" I asked.

"They just don't let him function."

"Function how?"

"You know," she replied, suddenly drawing the line after having been so explicit all along.

"You mean he has trouble having an erection?" I asked gingerly, suddenly realizing that I had never spoken about sexual matters to an Englishwoman before.

"If it were only trouble that he is having, I could help," she replied, recrossing the line, "but he doesn't even try anymore."

Since shortly after their arrival here, Alton had not made any sexual advances to her. This was in such contrast to what had happened during their affair and immediately after their marriage that she finally questioned him about it. He told her that he had gone to a doctor (strange, he had not told me about that) as soon as they came to New York, that his blood pressure had been found to be very high, and that he therefore had had to increase the dose of one of his medicines. Both his desire and his erections had disappeared soon thereafter, and that was how he explained his newly acquired total lack of interest in sex.

All my life, I have in one way or another felt sorry for suffering women, or at least those who claim to be suffering. I was very careful not to jump to conclusions based on Valerie's story alone, especially because of this tendency of mine, but I was suspicious. Men lie about their sexual function all the time, usually to cover up what seem to them to be shameful inadequacies. But Alton's response, suggesting that his sexual function was fine, to my questions in this area had seemed genuine and unconflicted. What's more, he was taking a very small dose of reserpine, a blood-pressure-lowering drug then very much in vogue. Although I had seen even small doses reduce sexual potency in men, it was difficult for me to imagine that a minimal increase in the medication to the current tiny dose would so dramatically have reduced his sexual powers from good to nonexistent.

Besides, "Nobody's been complaining" had to be seen as a strange answer, unless it was just meant to be funny, but it added to my suspicions. I resolved to keep the Beale family situation in mind, and specifically to investigate Alton and his medication history further on his next visit.

I found out what I wanted to know sooner than that, though, because he was admitted to the hospital with a heart attack ten days later. At that time, I had admitting privileges at three hospitals. When Alton called one night complaining of chest pain that had awakened him from sleep and had not been lessened or stopped by nitroglycerin under the tongue, I suspected that he was having a heart attack. In those days, it was usually possible to find a bed in a hospital, and it was not necessary to keep patients stored in emergency rooms, as they are now. Naturally, I preferred to admit my patients to one of my two major teaching hospitals, but on that particular night neither one had an empty bed. My third choice, in which I just had admitting privileges but where I did not do formal teaching as in the other two, had mainly foreign interns and residents, a fact that at that time (but certainly not today) spoke for the slightly inferior quality of the hospital and of its teaching program. But a bed was available, there was no other practical choice, and I made arrangements for Alton to be taken there by ambulance.

Thirty years ago, there was no such thing as a coronary care unit, coronary artery surgery, or balloon dilatation of a blocked vessel. Patients with heart attacks were kept in the hospital for much longer than they are now, and a three-week stay was not at all unusual. Alton had no complications such as a disturbed rhythm, shock, or congestive heart failure, and, as a matter of fact, he was quite well during the entire hospitalization. It seemed to me that he had a personal relationship with every nurse, nurse's aide, and secretary on the floor, and that he was easily the most popular patient of the nursing unit and probably of the entire hospital. Valerie visited every evening after work and stayed for as long as they let her. She brought him special foods, made sure that he got his usual evening cocktail, and entertained him, in that droll English way, with imitations of some of the people in her office. Sometimes she seemed a little embarrassed when she saw me as I came by on my evening rounds. I understood why, of course. After all, she may well have felt guilty about complaining so bitterly to me about her husband such a short time before this terrible thing had befallen him!

I saw Alton twice a day, as was my custom with patients who had had heart attacks. Even though his recovery was unusually uneventful, by that time I had already been burned once or twice by a sudden turnaround in exactly this type of situation, so I continued to watch him very, very closely. On this particular day, my morning visit was at around seven-thirty, and I found Alton to be fine. In those early years of my practice, in addition to going to three hospitals, I had daily office hours and also held down a part-time job in a union clinic, so my evening hospital visits were sometimes delayed into the night. If the patient was sleeping, and nothing seemed to be wrong, I would not wake him. The act of seeing for myself that everything was all right satisfied me, however, and I could then go home feeling that, at least for the moment, all the bases had been covered.

It was around eleven-thirty P.M. when I came to check on Alton. The door to his private room, at the end of the hall, was closed. Hospital rooms cannot be locked, of course, because of safety regulations, so I was surprised when I sensed resistance when I pushed on the door. It felt as if there was a chair wedged up against it. As I began to push against the obstruction, I heard whispering, followed by the rustle of bedclothes, and then the sound of feet hitting the linoleum floor. The room had been dark, but the light from the hall now showed two distinct shapes, one on the bed, the other scurrying away from it. It was too late for me to quietly close the door, especially since I realized that the occupants of the room could easily see my outline backlit by the strong fluorescents in the corridor. At that moment, I had very mixed emotions. It seemed to me that I had walked in on a conjugal hospital room tryst between Valerie and Alton, and I was happy that the sexual silence between them was finally broken. Patients are always asking how soon they can make love after they are discharged from the hospital after a heart attack. The answer depends on the particular doctor's judgment and not on any scientific rule. But sex while still convalescing in the hospital? I was strongly against it, though admittedly mainly out of medical prejudice. I just could not help but disapprove of an activity that subjected the recently damaged heart muscle to heart rates of 160 beats per minute and to systolic blood pressures over 200.

But it did not turn out to be Valerie who was sitting on the bedside easy chair wrapped in a blanket, face flushed, lipstick just a vestige, her bra and panties lying at her feet like faithful little dogs. It was Sophia, the resident on Alton's case since his admission to the hospital!

One of the fringe benefits of being in medicine is that you can always take refuge in the basics. So I immediately resorted to my concern for the patient, casting aside worries over cosmic issues such as faithfulness, passion, deception, and the like. My first impulse was to go over and examine Alton, to check his pressure and heart and lungs, as we did after a patient had had a Master's Two-Step, the primitive forerunner of today's sophisticated stress tests. But I was reluctant to intrude on his privacy, to touch him so soon after his obvious exertions with Sophia. As a matter of fact, I wanted to get away from there as quickly as possible, to keep everyone's embarrassment to a minimum. Observation of the patient, looking at him carefully, has always been held in high esteem by good clinicians. Just this once, I confined myself to this method of evaluation, leaving aside the familiar smelling and listening and palpating. Alton's face had a healthy color; he was not clutching his chest, and his respiration appeared normal. He was not sweating (at least his face wasn't), and although he looked appropriately disturbed, he was obviously not in distress. I was satisfied that he had had no evident untoward effects from the evening's activities. What's more, since the resident on his case was sitting there undressed, except for a blanket, it was hard to ask her to do an electrocardiogram right then and there. So I muttered something about seeing them in the morning and went home.

By the time I arrived in the hospital early the next day, I was already being paged. Sophia wanted to see me, and we met for breakfast in the cafeteria. She was in her forties, about ten years older than I, and had been a dermatologist in Greece before emigrating to the United States several years before. She was dark haired and very lively, and was pretty despite, or maybe because of, a tendency of her right eye to wander. Yet she had never looked particularly coquettish to me, and I suspected that what had happened on the previous night was due at least partially to Alton's increasingly obvious seductive powers. State law required a certain amount of American training before the licensing examination could be taken, and that was why she was in the program, despite her age and experience. I had always been embarrassed by the fact that she was basically my student, even though she was significantly older. She had put me at ease right from the beginning of our relationship, though, and we had become good friends.

130

Playing God

We did not waste any time in discussing the previous night's events. I immediately assured her that what had happened would remain confidential and that she had nothing to fear from me as far as telling the hospital authorities was concerned. I also told her that my chief concern was for the welfare of the patient and that she should have known better than to let him subject himself to this kind of stress so soon after a myocardial infarction. She admitted in turn that one thing had led to another, and that she had not used her best judgment, but that the bottom line was that she was in love with Alton, that despite everything the experience had been wonderful and satisfying, and that she definitely intended to continue seeing him.

Ethically, I was in a strange position. I knew that she would ultimately be another victim of my patient's compulsive behavior toward women, but I could not reveal to her what had been told to me in confidence by Valerie. The only thing left for me to do was to turn into a wise old bird with this lady whose experience in life was obviously much greater than mine and to warn her not to put her family or her career at risk for somebody who was "not only sick, but also married." This was pretty weak preaching, and I wished that I could have told her everything I knew about Alton in order to protect her. But I was so perplexed at this point that it took me a few more days to try to play God, although in a different setting.

A short time later, Valerie came to see me in my office on the day before her husband was to be discharged from the hospital. It was, of course, now obvious to me that Alton was not impotent and that the story he had told Valerie was just that, a story. It seemed to me that he had probably been having an affair with someone since shortly after their arrival here and that that was the reason for the abrupt termination of his sexual contact with his wife.

I was prone to feeling sorry for Valerie, as I have already

said. But the trick that Alton was playing on her made me indignant as well. The compassion I felt, together with my anger, pushed me into trying to rearrange Valerie's life—without her permission, naturally, and for reasons I was the only one to know.

As we discussed Alton's diet, activities, and medications, the question of sexual activity came up, as expected. As I had planned, I told her, keeping the facts as vague as possible, that her husband's illness and the medications that he had to take would, for the time being at least, keep him impotent. I felt safe in telling her this lie because it seemed obvious to me that, if Alton already had an affair with someone else, and the hospitalization had added Dr. Sophia to his harem, it was very unlikely that he would resume sexual relations with his wife in the near future. But then I suggested something to her that I had also planned and that since that time has seemed completely indefensible to me. I advised, not in so many words but with the meaning unmistakable, that she should find a boyfriend, someone who would satisfy her sexually but who would not break up her marriage!

I felt pleased that I had come up with such an eminently fair solution to Valerie's problem. Even though I could not share my special knowledge of Alton's activities with her, I could at least right the wrong that he had done her! The warm feeling of self-satisfaction I was experiencing was very short-lived, though. Valerie was repelled by my suggestion to find an outlet for her sexual frustration. "You don't understand me at all, Dr. Berczeller," she said, somewhat primly, I thought. "I love Alton, and if I can't have sex with him, I don't want it with anybody! Besides," she added, "I find that a curious suggestion for a doctor to make!"

My face became very flushed (it must have been bright red), and I considered myself properly told off. She disapproved of me because of the advice I had given her, which she obviously thought was improper. But at that moment, I disapproved of myself for an entirely different reason. I had tried to play God, to move my patients around like so many chess pieces on a board, and I felt ashamed. Yet I did not regret sympathizing with Valerie, who was being fooled repeatedly by a highly manipulative and sexually compulsive individual. I did regret doing what was so obvious to me by then, and that was, in my own way, to attempt to be as manipulative as Alton.

Alton retired soon after his heart attack, and the Beales moved to one of those places like Sea Island or Hilton Head. Years later, Valerie came to my office one day, unannounced. I had seen Alton's obituary a few months before, and as I was telling her of my regret at his death, I noticed that she had a very angry look about her.

"All these years I have wondered about that ridiculous suggestion you made to me, and I have always thought that it was because you were young and inexperienced," she began, almost magnanimously. "But ever since I found out that Alton was having an affair with his second wife while he was telling me that he was impotent because of the medication, I began to realize that he had put you up to it."

"Put me up to what?" I asked.

"To suggesting that I get a boyfriend so that Alton could conveniently take his business elsewhere," she replied, much more fluent in the American idiom than in the past.

I was at an enormous disadvantage. Exactly because of the confidential nature of the doctor-patient relationship, I still could not tell her what I had witnessed in Alton's room that night. The episode with Sophia had alerted me to Alton's dishonesty toward his wife, and that was why I so misguidedly had tried to help her. To be accused of being a tool of Alton's in some plot against his wife was very painful, even after all those years. All I could say to her was that Alton and I had never discussed *any* of his previous wives and that I had only been his doctor and never his instrument.

I don't know whether she believed me or not, but I was unhappy all over again about the error I had made such a long time before. By this time, though, I had already heard the joke I mentioned earlier, and my latest unpleasant meeting with Valerie had made me more convinced than ever that even if God can play doctor, doctors should never be so presumptuous as to play God.

Clinicians are first-class scroungers. They are never too proud to take whatever little bits of information may come their way and squirrel them away in their memories, the cookie tins and little sewing boxes of the brain. These modest treasures, the equivalents of old buttons and pieces of string, come in handy sometimes as shortcuts to understanding patients and their illnesses; so *experience* and *intuition* may just be fancy words for what we do when we polish up old impressions and apply them to new situations.

It was my custom to check my waiting room several times a day just to make sure that all scheduled patients were accounted for and that there were no possible victims of the office bureaucracy sitting there, completely ignored. One day, I noticed a middle-aged couple on one of the settees, and I had an immediate feeling that I knew a lot about them. The way they clung to each other, holding hands and whispering, the man's coat and hat on the woman's lap, reminded me of married people I had known, so dependent only on each other that there was no room for children, and who focused on their mate's well-being to the exclusion of the rest of the world.

It turned out that I was not far off the mark. The Kellers, Stephanie and Sidney, ran a mom-and-pop operation, a clipping service for individuals and organizations who wanted to keep track of what was being written about them. They were childless, as I had suspected, and commuted by bus every day to their office on lower Broadway from their house in central New Jersey. She was very short, with a curved spine and spindly legs. He was tall and thin, with a furrowed face and a startled, worried look that was, from what I could see, a permanent fixture. At first it was difficult to get an accurate history, because both of them tried to give me information about Sidney's condition at the same time. In these situations, I have found it helpful to suggest that a spokesman be appointed, and sure enough it was Stephanie who was elected to do the talking.

Sidney was then sixty-two and had had diabetes for thirty years. Despite large doses of insulin, his blood sugar was not well controlled, and it was often too high or too low. Fortunately, his vision had been spared so far, but the disease had affected his blood vessels and he had already had two TIAs, or transient ischemic attacks, with temporary paralysis.

There was, of course, no question in my mind that Stephanie would be with us in the examining room. She helped him to undress, frequently stretching up to stroke his face, and then she sat down on the little examining stool and watched me intently as I did the physical. I did not find anything particularly surprising, except that his blood pressure was 180 over 100, evidently a new finding. So I gave him a prescription for an antihypertensive, rearranged his insulin dosage, and asked him to come back in ten days so we could discuss his results and check on his blood pressure and sugar.

About a week later, my service called me early one evening and asked me to call a New Jersey number, that it was an emergency having to do with Sidney Keller. I had spoken to Stephanie several days before, and she told me then that

Sidney's sugar had come down with the change in the insulin dosage and that he felt "stronger" with the new blood pressure medication. At first, the line was constantly busy, par for the course, as I have said before, for emergency calls. When I finally got through, it was not, as I had expected, Stephanie on the telephone. There was a constant loud wailing in the background, making it more difficult for me to hear the lady on the other end. From what I could understand, though, Sidney had suddenly died, and Stephanie had called her to come right over. When I asked her if she was a relative, she answered in a puzzled way that she wasn't even a friend, let alone a relative, that they had met on a cruise two years ago and had not seen each other since, even though they lived not far from each other. The wailing evidently belonged to Stephanie, and when I asked to speak to her, it took a while for her to come to the telephone. She was sobbing terribly, but after a few minutes she became slightly calmer. At first we spoke of what had happened that evening. She told me that, during dinner, Sidney suddenly complained of a very severe headache. He lost consciousness almost immediately after that, and then stopped breathing. It sounded to me as if he had ruptured a blood vessel in his brain, and I assured her that nothing could have been done to save him, even if, for instance, he had been in a hospital, or if he had had medical attention right away.

She seemed satisfied with my explanation, but there was something else on her mind. "Doctor," she said, "Sidney's wish was to be buried in England, which he always loved. Last year, we bought a double plot in a cemetery in Sussex, and as soon as I bring his body there, I'm going to make funeral arrangements for both of us, and then I'll kill myself." The words were dramatic, but the way in which she spoke was so matter-of-fact that I had to believe that she was serious. She and her husband had made the impression on me of people who planned carefully, so I doubted very much that this was just some hysterical outburst.

I knew that it would take quite a few days for her threat, or really, rather, her promise, to become a reality. The first thing to do was to try to help this poor woman in her immediate distress, so I prevailed upon her acquaintance-become-very-reluctant-next-of-kin to take her to her home overnight and to give her five milligrams of the Valium that had, in the meantime, been found in the Keller medicine cabinet. Stephanie and I agreed to stay in very frequent touch over the next day or two, and that we would see each other soon.

When she came to my office at the end of that week, she was composed. Although she was no longer wailing or sobbing, it was clear right away that she had not changed her mind about her transatlantic plans. I had, of course, realized from the very beginning, from the way that they sat, almost merged into each other, in my waiting room, that the Kellers were one of those couples who had finally become inseparable twins. "I can't live without him (or her)" is a romantic declaration we have all made or heard at one time or another. I would not have been surprised if Stephanie had explained her intention to kill herself on this basis, but what she said was much darker and more final: "I can't let Sidney be in the grave all by himself. I was always with him, and soon I'll be with him again."

Ever since she first told me of her intentions, I had been at a loss about what to do, and the conversation in my office just reinforced my dilemma. Talking about committing suicide is not a crime, as far as I knew, so calling the police was not justified. She had appeared perfectly normal, though very anxious, when I first met her, and her grief at her husband's sudden death was not out of the ordinary. Yet the suicide–double funeral idea was not only outside my experience, it was the only time I had ever heard of anything remotely similar except for the custom of certain Indian sects for the wife to throw herself upon her husband's funeral pyre. I had passed the problem by David, a psychiatrist whose opinion I valued very much and with whom I often discussed situations in my practice that were on the borderline between psychiatry and medicine. He offered to see her, but I knew she would never go to a psychiatrist, especially not now. Yet from what I told him of her, he thought that she was very likely not psychotic, and that what she was planning to do appeared to make perfect sense to her.

If I could only have spoken to some of their relatives! A large family closing ranks around one of its desperately sad members can sometimes reverse the most melancholy plot for self-destruction. To my knowledge, though, the Kellers had no close relatives. Otherwise why would she have called a casual acquaintance for help during what was probably the gravest moment of her life?

Could a clergyman make the difference? Was she observant enough so that he could prevail upon her not to do what only God is entitled to do, and that is to take away life? Even more, could I help? What could I tell her in order to change her mind? And was it even right to try to dissuade her from doing something that, in her mind, reinforced her bond with her husband? And if I could convince her not to do it, wouldn't she be even more miserable in the future than she was now?

I went through the motions, because my commitment is to try to keep people alive, whatever the cost. She wasn't interested in psychiatry, family, religion, or, as she stated very courteously, in what I had to say. We parted cordially after she promised, "You'll hear from me." I never saw her again.

She was true to her word. About two weeks later, I received a letter postmarked "London." For a while after, I was able to repeat the contents by heart, but now I just remember the gist of what she said. She thanked me for what I had tried to do to keep her alive but wrote that by the time I received her letter she would be resting very close to dear Sidney in the English soil they had both come to love so much. She was sorry that our relationship had been so brief, but said that the fact that I had at least seemed to understand what was pulling (not pushing) her in the direction she finally took had given her peace of mind.

For a doctor to play God is not only implausible; the very idea is infinitely complicated. If I had used the information confidentially given to me by Stephanie that she was going to kill herself, and by various maneuvers kept her from going through with it, would I have been playing God then? Yet didn't I play God by, in essence, letting her kill herself because I had not put massive obstacles in her way? It's quite possible that, in this very special situation, wherever I turned I played God. But I never felt that I had control over her situation. I just held off from forcing things either way, something that made me more of an instrument. And I'm willing to live with that.

Should doctors, under proper legal safeguards, be allowed to hasten a patient's death? This is a burning issue, not only here but in Europe as well. It is not just the lunatic fringe on the patients' as well as the doctors' side that supports the idea, but people in the mainstream also, and there is no doubt that everyone means well. Yet most people, and the societies of which they are a part, are at least conflicted about the extreme nature of yet another final solution, this time to illness.

But isn't it a paradox that we are talking about sweeping some people out of this life while we expend huge effort and large amounts of money on keeping others alive longer and longer? I am aware that the two groups are not similar. The ones who want to die, and whom we are considering killing, are mainly the "goners," the ones who were so sensitively called "incurables" in the old days. They are the rejects of modern medicine, whose lives have been so devastated by pain, or deterioration of body parts, or whatever, that life's very definition has been downgraded into that of mere existence.

The other ones, who used to die on schedule, when their disease told them to die, what about them? They are yesterday's "goners," and maybe tomorrow's, too, when they will have reached the end of the line. But isn't it only right that we should pull out the stops for them today and keep them with us as long, as happily, and as comfortably as possible?

Of all the living wills I have seen, the copies of which I have put in the patients' charts like so many insurance policies against prolonged suffering, I have never seen one in which a request was made by a patient that he actually be put to death under certain circumstances. Certainly the standard desire expressed was to avoid unusual efforts to prolong life needlessly, but this is a much more acceptable, passive way to invite death. Life is not cheap, whichever way you slice it, and most of us have a horror of killing or being killed.

What do people who accept even the most degraded imitation of life have that those who request the sure, clean release from suffering that death is do not? It is hope. There are very few of us who can live without hope, and it is the last thing we cling to, even in (or maybe especially in) desperate circumstances. The faint glimmer of a possible last-minute reprieve means more to most of us than a sure bright light at the end of our last tunnel. Whenever one of my patients, obviously expecting to be kidded out of it, said, "I can't wait to die, I'm suffering so," I would invariably reply, "Life's the only game in town, so hold on to it. You're going to have a long time to be dead!" I meant it then, and I still do, for myself included. Most people want to live at whatever cost, and it is the exceptional person who is so lacking in hope that he has the courage to make plans for his own death.

My wife's Uncle Bill was part of this minority. My mother-in-law and one of her sisters were widows, and another two had never married, so only her sister Rose had a living husband. He was the proverbial rooster and ruled his hen yard with an iron hand. When I first came into the family, he had for years been its president and treasurer, in charge of anything from cemetery plots to savings accounts, and I was given to understand that he had a vile, unpredictable temper. His gas station in New Rochelle was legendary. The service was courteous and the mechanical work was reasonable and reliable, so he always did good business and was able to make side investments in real estate as well. What's more, he hadn't gotten those strong arms and that weather-beaten face for nothing. The station was open seven days a week, and I had heard through the grapevine that family members, even girls and day visitors, would be pressed into service pumping gas when things became unusually busy.

In those days I also had sudden rushes of anger, in other words, a temper, and I understood later that the initial meeting between Uncle Bill and me was the subject of much concern for my mother-in-law and her many sisters. I don't know what they expected, but our famous tempers did not venture out all afternoon. We liked each other immediately, especially since I had no designs on either the presidency or the treasury of the family. I was given to understand, though in not so many words, that I was being appointed a consultant to Uncle Bill, and therefore to the family at large. At that time, I preferred to believe that my thirty-year-old's bravado and charm had impressed him immediately. Years later, I realized that, instead, my profession had given me my initial boost, since Uncle Bill belonged to a generation that still unconditionally respected doctors.

Soon after our wedding (Uncle Bill had given my wife away) he came to my office for a checkup, and from then on he was my patient. What's more, some of his customers saw me as well, their trust in him obviously even extending to medical matters. About ten years later, Rose, his wife, died, and a while after that I became his confidant in the ever-touchy matters of later-in-life dating and sex with not always understanding strangers. He finally met Ida, a blond widow of about his age, and a couple of months later, he married her.

One day he came in with a story of recent upper abdominal pain, together with some weight loss. I felt a mass in his abdomen, and the x-rays suggested enlargement of his pancreas. At surgery, he was found to have a pancreatic cyst that looked benign, and we were all very relieved. Soon after that, he sold his business and his house and moved to Florida.

It turned out that we had been fooled. Some cancers of the pancreas form cysts, and this was one of them. He had been reoperated in Florida because of a return of the mass, and the definite diagnosis was made there. My wife and I went to see him there, after his discharge from the hospital. He had bought a place in one of those retirement complexes in West Palm Beach. It was called Leisure Village, Heritage Village, or something like that. The buildings were two-story and made of tan cement blocks, with the upper apartments approached by a sort of gangway. His was on the ground floor and consisted of what looked like several motel rooms tied together by a narrow hall. We found him in the tiny bedroom, lying on his side in the fetal position, probably the most comfortable one in view of his abdominal mass. He had always been a trim man, but now he was very thin and it was obvious that he had lost a great deal of weight in a short time.

There was no use playing games. I knew that he knew the truth, so we were spared the lying little games that well-meaning doctors play with their patients. At first, we spoke of the family. Since his illness, and especially since his move to Florida, I had more or less taken over his duties. But by then, three of the sisters were dead, so my reign was only over my mother-in-law and one of her remaining sisters. His former kingdom was much diminished, and therefore I had little to report to him. We tried several more conversational gambits; his own children were usually the cause for fifteen or twenty minutes of angry monologue, but nothing doing this time. We finally got to the inevitable, and it was really a relief for us both.

He came right to the point. "How long have I got?" he asked, in the same tone he must have used when he asked a customer how much time he had to do a greasing and an oil change.

"It's hard to say," I replied. "Talking about how much time you have left is for the movies!"

"Bullshit, but forget about that. I want you to give me something to end it while you're here; you're here for the weekend, aren't you?

"Bill," I said, "I can't just give you something! People think that doctors—"

"Bullshit again," he replied, raising himself on one elbow. "Those old ladies in the family have finally made an old lady out of you!"

I was glad that I had made him angry; I wanted to see that self-righteous anger erupt just one more time. But even in this he was so diminished that he reminded me of one of those real-looking guns that pop a cork out of the barrel when the trigger is pulled. We finally agreed to talk about it again the next day, and I promised that I would keep my mind open.

The next day, there was no small talk. As soon as I came into the bedroom, he began his plea to die. "Ida's miserable, and she can't help me. I'm helpless, I can't sleep at night because I can't find a spot for myself. I'm just a bag of bones. What good am I to anybody?"

I just couldn't say good-bye to him, obviously for the last time, without giving him a little encouragement. Usually we comfort people by suggesting that they are going to live. In this case, I held out the hope for death by lying to him that I would try to arrange, at my hospital in New York, what he was asking for.

I had never kissed him before—he was not the kissing type—but I did now. My wife did the same. I promised to keep him informed, and we left. After my return to New York, I called him every day and urged him to take as much pain medication as he could. He must have seen through my lie, because he never again spoke about a rapid death. Yet he got what he wanted; by the weekend after our departure, he died at the favorite witching hour of cancer patients, around five or six o'clock in the morning.

I am sure that he was very disappointed with me. We had been so close, he must have thought, and he had never asked me for anything, ever. What's more, he must have been angry that I put him off instead of doing something he thought should have been easy for me, like giving him a drug overdose.

What Bill didn't take into account (and at that stage of the game, why should he?), and what is not generally known, especially since it is talked about so little, is that most doctors cannot conceive of killing a patient, whatever the circumstances. Of course, it is against the law as well, obviously a major deterrent, but it seems to me that even if mercy killing were to become legal under certain conditions, few physicians would be willing to actually do the job. It is hard to break, even occasionally, with the philosophy and the teaching and learning of a lifetime. Our whole thrust is to preserve life, so to do the exact opposite is unthinkable for most of us. Yet even before living wills came into vogue, many of us did not pull out all the stops in treating obviously terminally ill patients, and instead let them die peacefully. Is this, then, so different from legally pulling on whatever trigger is agreed upon and hastening the death of the same group? Yes, it is, because in the one case we are keeping the patients comfortable and, we hope, pain-free while waiting for the natural end to come, and in the other we are playing God, and in the process we presume to decide when life is to be stopped.

I do not doubt that legally sanctioned death for certain categories of patients is the wave of the future. I don't disagree with the idea, because it is certainly sometimes more humane to stop life than to let it continue. Yet I am terribly conflicted about the actual turning off of something that is the only thing we know. Society justifiably assumes that doctors will have a central role in mercy killing; after all, aren't we in the health and life business? But that's just it, we are in the life business, not the death business. Call it cowardice or, worse yet, passing the buck, but I don't believe that doctors should be the ones to execute the death sentence. With very few exceptions, we are one-trick ponies, and we know only how to go in one direction—and that is toward life.

Then who should do the job, if not the doctors? If thanatology is defined as the study of matters related to death, then maybe thanatology technicians (T.T.s) should be trained to become experts in this particular service. They would certainly not have any less regard for the precious nature of life than we do, they would certainly not be callous killers any more than we are, but at least they would not be carrying the same burden that causes such conflicts within us doctors.

But the patient, in easily the most crucial hour of his life, has the right to expect his doctor to be there. He is the one with the well-worn relationship with the patient, the one who can give the most comfort. But now he is also at an advantage, which is an advantage to the patient as well. Somebody else will give the injection, so the doctor does not carry direct responsibility for the patient's death. He is no longer trying to keep the patient alive, always a worrisome and problematic matter at best. He has succeeded in not playing God, but maybe he is a standby for Him, a reassuring presence in the patient's field of vision even as the light grows dimmer.

8

Other Opinions

CONSULTATIONS, or, as they are frequently called, second opinions, play a justifiably enormous role in patient care. An unusual physical finding, a laboratory test that doesn't make sense, an unexplained and unexpected worsening of the patient's condition, all these are certainly excellent reasons for asking another doctor to give his impression of what is going on. Ideally, this should be, as they say in the outside world, a "win-win" situation. That is, if the consultant has no additional diagnostic ideas or suggestions for treatment, then the patient, family, and referring doctor can all rest easy; everything that should be done is being done. And if the new broom comes up with a different approach to the patient's illness, then everyone in the original ménage à trois should feel relieved, because if there is change there is hope.

Then why doesn't it work out like this in real life? In my experience, nothing (except possibly the money issue) creates as much misunderstanding between patients and their relatives on the one side, and doctors on the other, as the if, the who, and the when of other opinions. Add to that the question of whether the consultant should replace the original doctor or whether he should at least be added to the team and you have the makings of a full-scale political struggle.

Some situations are less difficult than others, though. There are some patients who are afraid to ask for another opinion because they feel their basic doctor will interpret the request as a sign of lack of confidence in his abilities. They may not be all that sick and are frequently outpatients—let's say, of the kind who want another opinion before having surgery for severe arthritis of the hip. The patient is restless and anxious. He does not want to undergo an operation if it is not absolutely necessary, yet he does not know how to ask for help in finding out what to do. He has two choices: he can, at least temporarily, master his fear of the doctor and ask for a referral for another opinion, or he can quit the doctor before ever even finding out what the doctor's feelings are about having his patient seen by someone else.

Some may just be very timid, but there are many others who pick up something in the doctor's behavior that suggests that he disapproves of other opinions. There is no question that there are physicians who are very defensive, and it is insecurity that makes them consider consultation to be the same as "meddling" with their cases. Yet there are many others—usually, those who feel more secure about their handling of any particular situation—who are perfectly happy to do what the patient requests, if he would only make his wishes known.

It is often difficult for us to judge how anxious a patient really is and what he really wants. But if, though he is unsure about how the doctor will respond to his request, he has the courage to ask for something that is his right, then the doctor cannot refuse him. To do so would not only show insensitivity to the patient's needs but would also demonstrate incredibly bad judgment. Can a patient be blamed if, after having been refused access to consultation, he blames the worsening of his condition on the uncooperative doctor?

Of course, experienced physicians have a sixth sense about when their patients are beginning to think about wanting another opinion. It is something we pick up in the patient's face, an unusually thoughtful look, perhaps, or his newly self-conscious manner, but it is something subtle, something our instincts pick up. To offer consultation then, early enough to spare him embarrassment, makes the patient happy and, in the bargain, makes the doctor look good.

Most of the time, though, many of the circumstances surrounding other opinions are not straightforward. Even if it is relatively easy to solve the problems between the too modest patient and the reluctant doctor, the majority of situations are more complicated. The patients are usually quite sick, and it is not just a question of whether or not to undergo an elective operation. Their families at the same time have a sense of helplessness, and already have a foreboding of the chill of guilt they will feel if it turns out that they had not been "doing enough." What's more, the doctor has to decide (for the umpteeenth time in his career) exactly what the limits of his capabilities are.

Most patients do not understand that it is in their interest to get the most out of any one particular doctor and that "topping off" with any number of others is not necessarily to their advantage. There is really no replacement for the amount of imagination, enthusiasm, and, most important, concern that can be squeezed out of a conscientious physician who, though he feels equal to the clinical situation, also feels pushed into a corner by it. This is why the timing of other opinions is so critical. Unless the patient's situation is immediately life-threatening, the basic doctor has to be given a chance to set the scene properly. By that I mean that it is his job to give a name to what looks like a random, confusing set of symptoms and findings. To do this, though, requires not only the ordering of appropriate tests but something else of crucial importance, and that is the continued observation of the patient. It is probably very hard for nondoctors to believe, but there is a logic and a rhythm to each illness. Some diseases take longer to identify than others, not because the doctor is slow or because he is not paying attention but because nature, which controls illness, is far from being under our complete control.

Patients and their relatives cannot be blamed for wanting to train all the guns available on the despised illness—and at the same time, to boot. Go tell a frightened family that you can't shoot sparrows with cannon! But there is a real case to be made for giving the doctor some maneuvering room before asking him to call a consultant or expecting him spontaneously to suggest one. Anyone who has been in medicine long enough has a few pet phrases that help him bridge the unavoidable gap between our thinking and that of our patients. "How can I ask somebody for a second opinion when I haven't even come up with a first one yet?" was one I utilized frequently when I felt that the idea of a consultation was pushed prematurely by patient or family, and sometimes it helped to give them a better understanding of what I was trying to do for them.

I first met Sharon Glass, a heavily smoking, highly nervous advertising executive, late one night in the emergency room. Her mother had called a little earlier (she had been given my name by Rita, a dear patient of mine), and when I heard that her daughter was in her twenties and had suddenly become short of breath, the first thought that came to mind was that she was throwing clots to her lungs. This is the kind of short-hand clinical thinking that we sometimes resort to, and when the combination of youth, female sex, and trouble with breathing was presented to what I call my "internal computer"—in other words, my judgment—the order that came back was the following: "She may be on birth control pills. Pulmonary emboli [clots to the lungs] are a known complication of these medications. Sudden difficulty in breathing is a serious symptom, even if your first thought is not correct, and she is not on the pill. Don't work through the emergency room staff! Go there yourself and make up your own mind about what's going on." Of course, judgment does not speak to the brain in such a formal, articulate way. Yet the thoughts and the order to go were quite clear, and this is why I found myself walking down First Avenue on my way to the hospital's ambulance entrance at two o'clock that morning.

It is usually not a good sign if, as happened this time, one (or, worse yet, several) of the emergency room nurses greet you with a dirty look while saying something like "That patient of yours is impossible! Where do you get them from?" The suggestion is that it is somehow your fault that nurse and patient are already not getting along and, what's more, that it is up to you to "straighten the patient out." So I was already prepared for trouble when I walked into the cubicle; and the scene that greeted me did nothing to lessen my apprehension. The atmosphere in the little room, the size of a large closet, was charged, as in the moments before a thunderstorm. The young woman on the stretcher, evidently Sharon, my new patient, was managing to take rapid, deep breaths while yelling through the oxygen mask that was fitted over her mouth and nose. What she was yelling exactly was not immediately clear, but the three other people in the room, obviously her parents and someone who was introduced as her boyfriend, appeared very agitated. Her father, who looked like a domineering type to me, kept ordering her, in a loud voice, to "calm down," while her mother, speaking more softly, pleaded with her: "Please, darling, don't breathe so fast!" Meanwhile her boyfriend, finally introduced as Keith, and at whom the worst of Sharon's yelling seemed to be directed, did not say a word but instead held her right hand (the left one had an IV placed near the wrist) with one of his own while pressing a wet towel onto her forehead with the other.

Doctors don't shoo families out of patients' rooms just to demonstrate their power. Often there is a very good reason for it, and usually it is because the doctor wants to be able to form his own impression of what is going on with the patient without interference by the family. Relatives, of course, mean well, but it is surprising how much information can be gotten from a patient if there is nobody there to either speak for him or to influence what he is saying.

After her parents and Keith stepped outside, as I had requested, Sharon quieted down quickly, but her rapid breathing continued. She appeared to be hyperventilating, a condition usually tied to stress, but I wanted to wait for the result of the blood gas, which had been drawn before the oxygen was started, before definitely making up my mind about the cause of her breathing problem. Her blood pressure was fine, her lungs were clear, and there was no obvious suggestion, in examining her legs, of any clots. She had been on birth control pills for many years and was a very heavy smoker. Aside from a chronic cough, however, she had never had any respiratory symptoms until that night, when she had become short of breath a little while after Keith had announced to her that he wanted to break up with her.

The blood gases showed no lack of oxygen, but did reveal a so-called alkalosis related to a loss of carbon dioxide. These results went along nicely with the hyperventilation I had originally considered and spoke very much against the presence of pulmonary emboli.

The paper bag treatment for hyperventilation is probably the cheapest form of therapy in medicine. Placing one over the patient's nose and mouth, and having him breathe into it, causes the carbon dioxide that has been lost because of the excessive breathing to come back into the lungs and then into the bloodstream. Sharon responded to the maneuver beautifully within minutes and began to breathe normally again, so I was soon able to remove her oxygen mask.

I am always happy when a patient turns out to have something trivial rather than the serious condition I had feared originally. So I felt very satisfied with myself as I brought Sharon's parents and the errant Keith back into the room, expecting them to be impressed with the transformation that had taken place in Sharon in just a few minutes. But the moment she saw Keith, she began to yell again, and this time I understood her, because she was not wearing the mask. "Traitor! Son of a bitch! I gave you everything, and you only make me miserable! Who is she? What's she doing for you that I didn't?" At the same time, her breathing speeded up again, and we were back where we started; father ordering, mother pleading, and Keith, probably so guilty and embarrassed that he could not speak, trying to hold her hands, as before. I was just about to explain what I had found out, that despite appearances we had found out what was wrong. At this moment, though, the chest x-ray, which had been done when she first arrived, was put up on the view box. I expected it to be normal. Contrary to popular impression, smoking in itself does not cause an abnormal chest x-ray, and certainly hyperventilation that can be stopped by breathing into a paper bag is not a sign of lung disease. Yet, to my astonishment, her x-ray looked terrible. It did not show just one little shadow that should not have been there. Instead, many thick, mean-looking streaks could be seen in both lungs. How could she have a normal blood oxygen and physical examination and yet have such a worrisome x-ray?

I explained my diagnosis of hyperventilation to them and, without going into it further, blamed it on some stress that she was going through. I was sure that the x-ray findings had nothing to do with the excessively rapid breathing, yet I couldn't say for sure what the cause of the abnormality was. My hope was that she might have sarcoid, a usually benign condition that is well known to cause horrendous-looking chest x-rays in patients who have no symptoms, and I shared this optimistic notion with the patient and her entourage. What I did not mention, though, was that spread of a cancer to the lungs, or a lymphoma, for that matter, can cause the identical picture. She was not getting worse, and had actually temporarily improved, and since the x-ray had probably already been abnormal for a while, I suggested that we try the paper bag again, give her some Valium to calm her down, and, as we like to say, wait and watch.

I thought my plan was reasonable, but this time it was her father who did the yelling.

"What is this sarcoid anyway?" he asked, managing to look both frightened and contemptuous at the same time. "My girl can't breathe, and there's something wrong with her x-ray. I don't think you know what she has! I want a lung man, what do they call it, a pulmonary person, a specialist in breathing!"

"Mr. Glass," I answered, "I never said that I knew exactly what was wrong with Sharon, at least with her x-ray, but I don't think it's the right time to call for a second opinion when we have so many more tests to do. It's too early in the game, and you're not going to find out much more than I'm telling you now."

"Call him," he bellowed, and then proceeded with the usual threats to call my chief, the hospital administration, and, what's more, to sue me if I did not immediately do as he asked.

As far as threats go, I, like most other experienced doctors, have been worked over by experts. That is to say, when there is a disagreement, we know almost to the minute when the cajoling or "straight talk" by patients and their families will stop and the threatening is about to begin. Yet it is not a question of fear for me, whether I give in or not. It is, rather, a matter of realizing that, after a certain point, it is useless to pursue a reasonable policy if the patient or his family is dead set against it. Education and explanations can go only so far, and the threats, although in themselves not so terribly frightening to somebody who has been around for a while, do mark the cutoff point.

It was four o'clock in the morning by the time I called the chest specialist who was on duty for the group with which I usually worked. The most junior partner, Alex, was the lucky man that night. He had been my trainee in internal medicine several years before and was still finding it difficult to accept my invitation to call me by my first name. It was obvious that he was startled by my call, since he must have realized from the story I told him that the patient appeared to be in no danger and that clarification of the chest x-ray abnormality could wait until later in the day. Yet when I told him that I had called at the insistence of the family, he came right over.

Doctors very rarely totally agree with one another in the evaluation of a case, but contrary to the impressions gathered from watching television, it is extremely unusual for the disagreements to be so crucial that the "chief of staff" has to be called upon to mediate. We basically operate by compromise, by consensus, as I like to say, and I have virtually never seen differences of opinion that are so drastic that a unified plan for the patient's care cannot be worked out. Yet I have always suggested, sometimes kiddingly, that only an odd number of consultants be called for a particular problem. In this way, embarrassing ties can be avoided and the tiebreaker is automatically built into the consultation process.

At the same time, I am offended, for all of us, by the frequently expressed suspicion of patients that we "cover up for each other." People do not understand. Medicine is not Watergate! We don't automatically side with other doctors and try to hide their mistakes. Almost all of us are very well aware of how thin the line is between success and failure in the handling of patients. Aside from the surgeons, who at least leave a scar to show that they actually did something, the rest of us have only opinions to dispense. And opinions are just that: not guarantees, not the gospel truth, just informed impressions. If they are all we carry in our now fictitious doctors' bags, does it make sense for patients to think that we would routinely corrupt the whole process by dishonestly supporting the misdeeds of other doctors?

Alex was obviously in a bind. On the one hand, he did not want to show disrespect for me by disagreeing with my view of Sharon's problems, but on the other, he wanted to prove himself. It is the rare consultant who does not at least find something he would do differently, one who completely agrees with how the case has been managed so far. After all, it is understandable that he wants to justify, in some way, having been called in in the first place. Besides, doctors, especially conscientious ones, are naturally competitive with each other. Alex, despite his youth and his regard for me, was no different, and he was bound to come up with a different handle on Sharon's clinical picture. She was no longer hyperventilating when he saw her, so he was less impressed with that diagnosis than I was. Sharon's longtime use of birth control pills impressed him to the point where he thought the normal blood oxygen did not necessarily rule out clots to the lung. Besides, he felt that the chest x-ray abnormality could possibly speak for an unusual pneumonia, which, in turn, might also have been the cause for the rapid breathing. I, of course, disagreed with him on both counts and had already given my recommendations to the family. His advice was to give Sharon blood thinners temporarily (in case she had thrown clots to the lung) and to start her on an antibiotic for treatment of the possible pneumonia.

Action, of whatever kind, is usually more reassuring to patients and their families than what we call "watchful waiting." Doing *something* distracts them, at least a little bit, from the anxiety they are entitled to feel, while doing "nothing," for whatever good reason, is discouraging. I was therefore not at all surprised when Alex's recommendations were accepted over my own. What he proposed was much more than I would

155

have done, but it was not in itself wrong, so I was able to reassure Sharon and her parents (Keith obviously did not have voting rights) that his was a reasonable alternative to my own suggestions.

By later that day, we were able to stop the heparin—the blood thinner—because a lung scan spoke strongly against the likelihood of clots in the lung. An ACE assay (a blood test) and a CAT scan of the lungs virtually confirmed the diagnosis of sarcoid, so the antibiotic was stopped, but not before Sharon had developed a huge drug rash that kept her in the hospital for an extra few days.

If a doctor makes the right diagnosis and the patient recovers, he is a hero. As a matter of fact, even if he makes the wrong diagnosis but the outcome is favorable, he is at least treated with kid gloves. The first time I saw Sharon in my office after her hospitalization, her parents were with her. Keith was nowhere in sight, and when I asked for him, Sharon rolled up her eyes and both her parents momentarily looked grim. Generally, though, there was good feeling in the air, and even Mr. Glass, the bellowing bull of a few days before, treated me with courtesy and, what was apparently unusual for him, warmth. I knew that praise was just around the corner and usually I don't mind it; after all, a good review never hurt anybody. Yet I did not want to go into the whole story of how Alex was wrong and I was right. I was not being unduly modest, but at that moment I felt more strongly about making a point than receiving compliments. Of course, it is possible that I was more unhappy than I realized about their going along with a novice like Alex rather than listening to me, but the outcome of our talk was very encouraging.

We doctors feel that we often do not get through to our patients, not so much when we are dealing with their illnesses but when we try to educate them. Cigarettes, excessive alco-

156

hol, and high-risk sex are all habits we try to discourage, but individual patients' responses seem awfully slow to us. Almost as long as I have been in private practice, I have tried to convey to patients how they can best help themselves by knowing how to deal with the doctor. I have refused to see patients who wore curlers to my office and have insisted on some kind of greeting like "Good morning" before the patient launches into a recitation of his problems. The reason for this attitude, which may well appear arrogant to some, is that I believe that the meeting between patient and doctor should always be as civilized as possible, with both parties looking and acting as well as they can. This dignifies the process; and it should be dignified, if we consider the serious nature of what patients and doctors discuss.

What I taught the Glass family, when not to ask for another opinion, may not appear all that important. Yet I don't know how we are going to get patients to understand us better, and at the same time get some kind of insight into how we operate, if we do not use every opportunity we get to explain the complicated nature of what we do. There is no reason patients or their families should instinctively know the right timing for a consultation, since in the world outside of medicine, *MORE + SOONER* = (usually) *BETTER*. This is just an example of why, in addition to finding out what is wrong with our patients and treating them accordingly, we have one other great obligation to them, and that is to educate them so they have the best possible chance to help themselves to be helped by us.

Premature consultation can be any number of things: wasteful, annoying, misleading, and even indirectly responsible for complications like Sharon's very itchy and ugly drug rash. Yet it is very rarely dangerous for the patient, which cannot be said, unfortunately, for consultation that is overdue, whether by hours or even by days.

* * *

Some years ago, a patient called and asked me to see his father, who had been admitted to a small private hospital in uptown Manhattan earlier that day. My patient had recently had a spontaneous pneumothorax, that is, an escape of air from a pocket in his lung into the chest cavity, and his father's shortness of breath and chest pain reminded him of the symptoms he had had. Mr. Russo, Sr., had been seen by a doctor on admission, who told the family that he was not sure of the cause of the symptoms, that the chest x-ray "doesn't show anything," and that further tests would be necessary. In the meantime, though, the patient's breathing had become more and more labored, and he had become very agitated.

Although I was not on the staff of the hospital, I agreed to come right over, since the situation sounded desperate. As I was driving uptown, I urgently tried to remember what I had been taught about the emergency treatment of tension pneumothorax, that is, air in the chest under such high pressure that it can push the heart out of place and ultimately cause shock and cardiac arrest. When I saw the patient a short while later, he was blue and barely breathing. I could not obtain a blood pressure, and he was virtually not responding. It was obvious that looking for the chest x-ray would be a waste of precious time. I tied a rubber finger cot around the outside opening of a large-bore needle (during my training, my surgical resident had mentioned a condom, but never mind) and then stuck the needle forcefully into the patient's chest on the side where, when I had briefly listened, I could hear no breath sounds at all. For a moment nothing happened. Just as I began to think that I might have been wrong in my diagnosis and that therefore the needle in the chest would make things worse rather than better, I heard a very welcome hissing sound, something like air escaping from a radiator valve. At the same time, the finger cot, acting like a balloon, began to expand and collapse with each breath the patient took. His lips and nail beds became pink almost immediately, and we were soon able to obtain a normal blood pressure. About an hour later, a chest surgeon who had been called put a drainage tube into the chest to remove the rest of the air, and within a few days the patient went home.

Afterward, I looked at the original x-ray, and it showed a large amount of air in the chest; in other words, he had had a pneumothorax all along. The film was very dark, though, and that was why the presence of air was missed when the x-ray was originally looked at. I sometimes like to tell this story, especially since general internists like me rarely get the chance to do anything dramatic with their hands. But what is really important about it is that it illustrates the need for prompt consultation if the clinical situation is unclear to the original doctor, and especially if the patient is getting worse. Mr. Russo's doctor was, of course, negligent as well, since he did not watch his patient carefully, and as a result the family had to take the matter of consultation into its own hands. Yet, negligent or not, if he had called for another opinion early on, I am sure that a consultant would have made the right diagnosis, thus sparing the patient the terrible experience of near death, as well as my last-minute makeshift heroics.

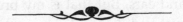

Experienced doctors have a sixth sense about when to call for consultation. I usually ask for help when I need somebody else's specific knowledge in diagnosis or in treatment to round out my own. Occasionally it turns out to be a more intimate process, though, and that is when I fear that the patient is going to die and I am not at all sure why. At those times, it comforts me to be able to go through the whole story once more with someone I trust, to try to justify what I have done so far, and to hope (in vain, usually) that my consultant will come up with something, anything, that will stop my patient's downward slide.

Who should be the one to give another opinion; in other words, who is an appropriate consultant? Nowadays in the United States, obtaining a second opinion in the case of a sick patient is the rule rather than the exception. As a matter of fact, medical insurance companies require a second opinion for certain procedures. Until about the mid-1960s, problems in internal medicine were handled mainly by "diagnosticians," that is, general internists of a higher caliber of training, who, after a thorough review of the case, made their recommendations and then did not come back unless they were asked to because of some new and drastic change in the patient's condition.

In the last twenty-five years, though, subspecialists (cardiologists, gastroenterologists, hematologists, and the like) have taken over the role of the diagnostician, and general internists have slipped a notch to where they mainly request consultation rather than provide it. At least a significant part of the medical profession is under the impression—the wrong one, as it happens—that CAT scanners and ultrasound machines are adequate substitutes for the skilled clinicians who, for instance, used to find lumps or diagnose leaky heart valves by using only their hands and ears. But that is my prejudice as an old-time general internist and diagnostician, and the reality is that, in our field at least, the subspecialists are doing most of the consulting. In other specialties, the generalists are still being asked to give opinions, but the call is increasingly going out for an "ear man," or a "knee expert," or somebody who has chosen the menopause as his field of expertise, leaving the rest of obstetrics and gynecology by the wayside.

I don't mean to imply that being seen by somebody who has focused, in his training and practice, on a particular area or problem is bad for the patient. On the contrary, specialized knowledge can cut through a lot of the red tape that surrounds both diagnosis and treatment, which is, of course, of great benefit to the patient. *How often* the services of a superspecialist are required is another question, however, and I will talk about that a little later.

Subspecialists in any field get pretty much the same training, read the same journals, and go to the same meetings. Does that have to mean, though, that individual qualities have to be thrown out the window? Just as I believe that patients have the right (not just the privilege) to have a personal relationship with their doctors, I think that consultants have to be picked for their human traits as well as for their qualifications. There is an unfortunate tendency nowadays, especially on the part of the residents, to call for "a GI consult," "a hematology consult," and the like, without knowing, or caring, who finally shows up. This kind of push-button approach lends an impersonal note to the consultation right off the bat. Is it any wonder, then, that the "consultant in the box," picked by the luck of the draw, is liable to focus on the illness at the expense of the total patient? And is it really surprising if, when the patient receives the bill, the following message is sent back: "I don't remember who you are. If you want to get paid, speak to the guys who sent you in the first place!"

It is hard to exaggerate not only the anticipation and the concern but also the hope that patients and their families feel when they know the consultant is on the way. For us doctors, another opinion may be just an additional piece to be put in the jigsaw puzzle of the patient's illness, but for them it is Judgment Day. What consultants have to say can be reassuring ("The angiogram looks good. You don't need surgery") or disastrous ("The bone marrow shows leukemia"), but *how* they say it, the human way in which they give their opinion, is much more important than even the news itself.

My father once told me something one of his professors in medical school said almost seventy years ago: "There are many doctors but few physicians." Any consultant who ever left my patient and his family hopeless or confused—in other words, who was so busy or emotionally out of touch that he did not give them anything to hold on to—was never called by me again. Most of medicine is not all that complicated, and it is not hard to find people with the technical expertise necessary to give up-to-date advice for many different conditions. But giving patients even a tiny bit of yourself, along with some hope, while remaining honest and straightforward, is an art that, in the long run, is at least as important as the science we find so much easier to peddle.

There is a dark side to this whole consultation issue, though, that bothers me very much. On the one hand, patients claim that they are seeking other opinions, when all they are doing is just "doctor shopping." On the other, doctors are both the culprits and the victims of medical care by committee, where the many have taken over the function of the one who used to take full responsibility for the patient. What both groups are really doing, though, is to exploit and to cheapen a traditional and respected process in which any number of doctors, when it was really necessary, put their heads together in a sincere attempt to pull the patient out of trouble.

First of all, what's wrong with doctor shopping? Isn't going to any number of doctors and asking them what they think of your problem the same thing as being sent by your doctor for other opinions? No, because patients often do not have the judgment to decide who is competent to advise on what problem. They will thus frequently find themselves seeing people who have nothing more to offer than their original doctor, or possibly even less. This, of course, goes completely against the whole basic idea of consultation, where it is hoped that someone with a special viewpoint, usually gained from advanced training and experience, will be able to help solve the patient's problem.

What's more, "doctor shoppers" are easy prey for practitioners who exploit patients' obvious anxiety and subject them to needless tests and expensive treatments. Besides, running from doctor to doctor is a good way for the patient to put off a dreaded diagnosis, since the workup is usually started all over again each time the patient consults somebody new. In addition, the patient can manipulate his own case (which is obviously to his disadvantage), since he will not stop until he finds a doctor who will tell him what he wants to hear.

What a patient obviously needs is a rational doctor who, though he is "pulling" for him to be well, keeps an eye on reality. He is there to protect the patient from fads, from unproven theories or treatments, and most of all, from the understandable yet often risky misjudgments arising from the patient's anxiety.

Previous generations knew how serious illness can be and how long it took to get better, if that was what was in store for you. The tremendous progress in medical research of the last years has created the wrong impression. The idea of instant gratification, so widespread in our society, has also worked its way into medicine, so that many patients lose confidence if a definitive diagnosis does not arrive in a matter of hours and "relief" does not happen within one or two days. The truth is that disease is forever something to be reckoned with, and doctors, who know it best, are very wary of it, as we would be of a dangerous and unpredictable animal. The most important thing for patients to realize is that doctors are not magicians. Leaving one, and especially one who has a good track record with you, and going to "a wonderful doctor" who "saved the life" of your friend is usually not the answer. The new magician will probably not cure you any more quickly, and the switch, in mid-illness, will probably cause even more delay in getting you better.

We all know what a committee is. It is a bunch of people who, it is hoped, agree on an issue and then speak as one. Yet who bears the responsibility when it is the patient who is at stake? A committee is, after all, just a lifeless object, so when something goes wrong it does not have the capacity to feel guilty or sorry. Yet the individual human beings who make up the committee are not obligated to feel responsible either, because everybody agreed, together, on the path taken.

I do not mean to imply that all medicine is practiced like this nowadays. But in internal medicine, as well as in certain other specialties such as cardiovascular surgery and neurosurgery, for example, it is not at all unusual for a hospitalized patient to have four or five doctors, each one seeing the patient every day.

What has brought us to this ridiculous state of affairs? Is it the need to practice "defensive medicine" because of the fear of being sued? I doubt it, because, if anything, the more doctors there are on any one case, the more the chances are that all of them will be legally involved in accusations of malpractice against one of them. Is it a financial matter? Maybe it is, to a small degree in some instances, because, after all, there was until relatively recently very little control over the number of doctors who could be reimbursed for the treatment of any one patient. In this way, a doctor could even be just marginally involved in the care of many patients and still receive a fee for each of his visits.

Yet I am not "covering up" when I say, at least in my personal experience and after years of a very interested overview of how medicine was practiced around me, that money is not at the root of this very revolutionary change in how many of us handle patients.

I think it has much more to do with our increasing timidity and self-consciousness. In the past, for a doctor to take full responsibility for his patient came, as they say, with the territory. I don't know how our medical ancestors felt about carrying this burden, but I am sure they realized they had no choice. Courage has always been expected of doctors; otherwise how could they possibly, over the years, have given little bits of it to their patients, especially in those days when they had very little else to contribute? It takes more than just superficial bravado to take care of a child with croup, to cut into a virgin abdomen, or to make the heart stop during cardiac surgery. Suddenly finding yourself treating a wheezing patient with pulmonary edema (water on the lungs) at home, as happened to me a few times during my moonlighting days, quickly either uncovered whatever courage you had or made you realize that all you could tolerate emotionally was to become a medical bureaucrat.

A few things have happened in recent years, though, that have made a great deal of difference in what doctors expect of themselves. First of all, because of recent discoveries, we have become even more aware than ever of how complicated the machine we are working on really is. It is as if the family car we have been driving for years turns out to have been atom-powered all along. The tendency, then, is to throw up your hands a little bit, to feel increasingly insecure about your knowledge in anything but your chosen field, your subspecialty. The obvious solution is to team up with others who also feel unsure of themselves in anything but what they know best, and for all of you to try to replace the one doctor whose beat this used to be. The word has gone out to patients and other doctors alike: there are people available who can focus down on almost any clinical problem with a very high powered lens. So isn't it worthwhile to utilize them, rather than people who look less intensively at a larger area?

It is not just in the hospital, though, that patients are managed by committee. A few years ago, I saw a patient who had switched to me from one of the excellent subspecialists at my hospital. In New York City at least, and probably in most places where there is no scarcity of doctors, there is a constant ebb and flow to every physician's practice. Patients, it seems, are always leaving one doctor and taking up with another, so in the long run, the numbers of those who come and go cancel each other out in this game of medical musical chairs. Yet people's motives for coming and going are another story, and I was always interested in why patients left someone else and came to me instead. It turned out that it almost always had something to do with the other doctor's behavior and level of caring, according to the patients, and rarely with his competence. Being kept waiting too long, difficulty in reaching him, moodiness, and lack of warmth were the usual complaints patients were not at all reluctant to voice as soon as they met me. Yet what did my ex-patients say to their new doctors about me? Very probably the same things, I suppose. Of course, I cannot prove my theory in most cases, except for the times over the years when a colleague and I in a sense "traded" patients—that is, one or two of mine switched to him around the same time that several of his came over to me. While we exchanged medical information on the various defectors from our practices (a conversation about a patient's clinical picture can be a very valuable supplement to the release of his medical records), we usually also had a chance to compare notes about their reasons for leaving. Usually, the complaints of those who left were almost identical, whether they were moving away from him or from me! I do not doubt that these patients had at least some justification for what they did, but the real question is whether

Other Opinions

it helped them in the long run. The answer is very difficult to define. Just as it happens in divorce and subsequent remarriage to somebody not that different from the original spouse, the *illusion* of change is sometimes all that is needed to gain satisfaction in the new relationship. At other times, though, patients realize that they have only exchanged one doctor's faults for another's, as do, for that matter, the disillusioned participants in marriages listed under numbers anywhere from two on up.

Yet in this instance, the patient had not left his doctor out of dissatisfaction with him as a person. In addition, he had the highest regard for my colleague's skill, as he immediately told me on our first meeting. For the moment, I could not imagine another reason for his sitting across my desk from me, but things became much clearer when he said, "It was the way he practices that finally confused me and, frankly, tired me out!"

His former doctor is a board-certified gastroenterologist, which means that he is also certified in general internal medicine, as I am. He was therefore perfectly qualified to act as the patient's basic, or family, doctor. What he did, though, according to the patient, was to personally take care of only his complaints of gas and chronic constipation (in other words, problems within the scope of his subspecialty) and to refer him out for all other problems. For instance, when the patient had a dry cough for a few days that did not go away with cough medicine, he was referred to a chest specialist, who proceeded to do a complete physical and ordered sputum tests and a CAT scan of the lung for what sounded to me very much like a postnasal drip. On another occasion, the patient had a few days of pain with slight swelling of one of his ankles. He was promptly referred to a rheumatologist, who again did a complete examination, ordered many blood tests, and finally came to the conclusion that he had "a touch of arthritis."

This happened several more times, and finally he had had enough. Patients are often much more eloquent than we give

167

them credit for, and he put it really well when he said, "My intestine, my lungs, and my ankle got very thorough care. But what about me?"

It is not just a matter of skills. It is also a matter of availability. For decades now, there has been no real control over the number of specialists and subspecialists that have been trained. From time to time we hear what sounds reasonable to us, and that is that we need a lot more primary care doctors to take care of our population. But specialists have been turned out in numbers way out of proportion to our need for them for years, and it is understandable if we utilize them now that we have them anyway.

Patients know what is going on. The excessive specialization that has come about because our profession has not adequately policed itself has not been lost on the general public. Especially in urban centers, it is common knowledge that there is a subspecialist for almost anything. For instance, cardiology, which is a subspecialty of internal medicine, has its own sub-subspecialties such as cardiac catheterization, stress testing, cardiac echo, and so on. Thus, even a very well trained cardiologist may be passed over in favor of a sub-subspecialist in this ever-ongoing quest for the best, in this eternal spotlighting of ever-narrower areas of expertise.

But isn't specialization the wave of the future? How can our society not take advantage of the medical progress that we have all paid for and that allows us the privilege of having highly trained doctors evaluate even our most trivial complaints? The answer, which may well come as a shock to many, and especially to those in our population who want "only the finest," is that a very high percentage (I am reluctant to give an exact number because I cannot really prove it) of medical problems can be handled by one competent and conscientious doctor. And not only that, but oftentimes it is better for the patient if he is not subjected, at least right away, to an intense scrutiny of his problem. An experienced internist or family doctor knows when to turn on the heat in the investigation, but until then (if it turns out to be necessary) a more low key approach is much less frightening to the patient—and, what's more, is cheaper.

Occasionally, we see something with which we require help, and then it is very reassuring to both the patients and us that there is someone available, with the background of training and experience, who can come to our aid. But even if he sees the patient and gives us all an excellent second opinion, does he really have to overstay his welcome? Most of the time, it is really not necessary for him to keep looking over the shoulder of the original referring doctor. Instead, he should withdraw and come back again only if the need arises.

Naturally there are situations when the patient's situation is so critical, and so many organs are involved, that he deserves to have the full, frequent attention of several doctors, each specially trained in some aspect of his problem. But this should be by far the exception, and not what is happening nowadays, when any number of doctors stick to a patient like flies to flypaper.

Excessive specialization has robbed otherwise well-trained doctors not only of some of their courage but also of some of their skills. It should be obvious to everyone that if they no longer use a part of what they learned, doctors will lose their feeling of competence in areas that have been denied to them because of the too easy availability of subspecialists. If they thus have one arm tied behind their backs all the time, who can blame them for calling a two-armed consultant more and more often, and earlier and earlier?

I haven't even spoken about the economic cost of this medical care by committee. It is hugely expensive for the government, the insurance companies, and, yes, us to have to pay for so many duplicated medical services. I personally hope that financial pressures will discourage something that is squarely the fault of us doctors—that is, a process that, although it has the word *consultation* attached to it, has more to do with exploitation of the system than with providing rational, up-to-date medical care for as many of our citizens as possible.

We need more family doctors and fewer specialists! Let's train the doctors who are the patients' court of first resort as well as we possibly can and give them the responsibility that is appropriate to their education, interests, and experience. At the same time, it is more reasonable and economical by far to have a relatively small group of genuine specialist-consultants who are not in economic competition with the very doctors who refer patients to them. They can do us all the most good by practicing their specialty exclusively, rather than occasionally casting a timid foot into the often murky waters of family medicine.

Medicine is made stronger by the availability of other opinions. No doctor is so capable or all-knowing that he will not benefit, when it is necessary, from someone else's knowledge and experience. Consultations from well-trained and enthusiastic clinicians can only improve medical care. But if the process of consultation is cheapened by excessive utilization to the point where the consultant is a safety net while the referring physician has not even gotten off the ground, we will be encouraging exactly what we don't want. We will then have primary care practitioners of limited quality, and we will continue to train large numbers of specialists who, though well educated, are not qualified to take care of a large number of people on a daily basis.

9

Friends and VIPs

IS IT A GOOD IDEA for patients to become friends or friends to become patients? These things happen all the time, but the real question is whether friendship between doctors and patients ultimately works out to everyone's benefit.

To begin with, why do people start out with a professional connection and end up with a personal link? The reasons range from just plain social attraction and shared interests all the way to a calculated exploitation of "something special" that one or the other party has to offer. Friendship does have its conventions, but spontaneity is its driving force, so friends are allowed a lot of leeway in their behavior toward each other. Of course, we encourage friendly and easy contact with our patients, but the doctor-patient relationship has its formal side, and actual social friendship rarely enters into it. Yet the temptation is always there to either go along with a patient's suggestion to "get together like regular people" or to suggest to one patient or another to come to dinner sometime and to continue, in an informal setting, the fascinating conversation begun during an office visit. But what has to be understood is that what seems like a friendly attraction between people—of the kind, let us say, that began with a chance meeting on vacation or at a dinner party—is not so simple if the relationship originally started out with one individual bringing his concerns and complaints (with many fears attached to both) to the other.

Patients are not aware of it most of the time, but isn't it "reasonable" for some of them to want even more protection than the doctor can give them through his knowledge and experience, and for them to try to obtain, in addition, that extra bit of solicitude and intimate attention that is reserved for his friends? And even if they never have to draw on that reserve tank of special attention, isn't at least the fantasy of its existence reassuring for them?

In real life, though, this hope for extraordinary treatment can never be satisfied. Sooner or later, many patients who are at the same time their doctor's friends become resentful as they realize that if they wish to get better, friendship or not, they will have to depend only on what they were offered in the first place, the doctor's expertise. Worse yet, they are at a disadvantage if they feel dissatisfied with the care given to them by their doctor-friend. You can always tell any doctor off, if need be, but how do you comfortably tell him off if he just had dinner with you and your family in an Italian restaurant last Saturday night? At those times, you may well think back to the good old days when you had a friendly but ordered doctor-patient relationship and you hadn't yet gone together into that swamp of conflicting emotions and relations that is so characteristic of friendships.

What about the doctor? What is in it for him if he drops all or part of his objectivity in dealing with the patient, replacing it with the kind of concern reserved for the well-being of a friend? The double role of doctor and friend is bound to make things more difficult for him, since he cannot (and, of course, should not) stop feeling medically responsible for the patient, regardless of the change in the overall relationship. So why do doctors knowingly go into situations that may well turn out to be troublesome for them? They must feel it is worth it, either because of the obvious pleasure they get from the connection or because, consciously or unconsciously, they, too, have ulterior motives. Doctors know many people and meet new ones every day. Just as patients harbor fantasies of the advantages that can come from having more than just professional contact with the doctor, the reverse holds true as well. If a doctor has a patient who is a successful stockbroker, let us say, doesn't it "make sense" if he hopes that in some magical way his investments will be even better protected and more tenderly handled if the stockbroker is his *friend* and not only his patient? And if a doctor, as is the case with a former neighbor of mine, wants to impress his colleagues (and probably also wants to reassure himself that he really matters), what could be more effective than invariably having a smattering of famous artists and journalists, all of them patients, at his dinner table? In these situations, the battlefield promotion from patient to patient-friend works for everybody. The patients are reassured by their nearness to the medical power wielded by the doctor, and in the trade-off, the doctor gets what looks to him like an economic or social advantage.

But the doctor can also lose. As an example, I have sometimes found that patients want to be friends with the doctor so they can adequately (and safely) express their hostility, usually under the cover of "just kidding around." Andy Papp, a record company executive, had been my patient for several years when he suggested one day, at the end of his checkup, that we and our wives go out to dinner sometime. He seemed quite embarrassed, and quickly added that the thought had been on his mind for a long time but he had only recently gotten up enough nerve to make the suggestion. It was obvious that it had taken courage for him to open himself up to rejection on my part, so I immediately tried to put him at ease. We had often chatted about music as well as about sports cars, two particular interests of mine, in the past, and I had come to realize that his knowledge in both subjects was vast. Not only that, but he was personally very charming, and his wife, whom I had seen just once as a patient, had struck me as vivacious and intelligent. So I was very tempted, but what won me over was that I just could not subject him to a loss of face by saying no to him.

One of the problems that come up when the doctor-patient interaction takes on the added dimension of friendship is that the doctor possesses confidential information about the patient, so he always has to be very careful about what he says, even in the most relaxed social situation. What's more, he can never drop his guard and act out, on the basis of emotion, something that is, of course, acceptable in friendships unencumbered by professional responsibility. At the same time, though, the patient feels more and more comfortable in the role of a friend and loosens up in his behavior toward the once-feared doctor. This is exactly what happened with Andy. Over the next few years, we would see each other fairly frequently. It turned out that I had judged Andy and his wife correctly. They were very well informed, and besides, they were gracious hosts as well as gracious guests. Yet there was something that bothered me throughout our relationship and that invariably came up at least once in every evening that we spent together. At some point, and not necessarily within the context of the conversation, Andy would come up with a series of hostile remarks about doctors. At times, the subject of our financial exploitation of patients would be in the foreground: "At least a mugger takes all your money at once; with you guys, there's never an end to it!" At other times, there would be bizarre references to the sexual power doctors can exert with the examining finger or the proctoscope. There were other topics, too, but the theme ultimately always came down to the unfair advantage doctors take of the innocent, unsuspecting patient.

Andy's statements made me angry. It was not even what he said; I felt that it was unfair of him to use social occasions with me, a doctor, to pour out his hostility toward the entire medical profession. Or worse yet, was he a guest at my table and not too subtly expressing his dislike of me personally? Whatever his true feelings were, though, he was first of all my patient, so my professional obligation to him blocked any expression of the anger I felt. I admit it, I did not know what to do, especially since there were now four of us involved in the relationship. Obviously, I could not cancel our friendship while retaining him as a patient. On the other hand, if I fired him as a patient, that would automatically signal the end of the friendship as well. These measures somehow seemed extreme to me, especially since they would have victimized his wife, who was entirely blameless in this affair. So I let it slide, even though my usual tendency is to be very sensitive and touchy when I feel in the least badly treated.

We met again recently, very soon after I quit my practice. This was a first for me. I could say and do what I wanted because I no longer had responsibility for the Papps as patients. In other words, this was a purely social occasion, with no professional considerations lurking in the background, and it felt very good to be a private citizen again. I had hoped that Andy would finally stop his aggressive comments now that I was no longer his doctor, but at the same time I was also wishing that he would do it just one more time so I could, without guilt, tell him off. By the end of the evening nothing had happened, and I had already begun to congratulate myself on the patience and diplomacy—never my strong suits, I must admit—I had shown in not dismissing him as either friend or patient in the past. Yet I was disappointed as well, because it appeared as if I was not going to be able to take advantage of my newly found independence and express my stored-up anger at him. But at the last moment Andy ran true to form! Just as they were getting ready to leave, he said, with a big smile, "So now that you've quit and can't screw patients out of their money anymore, what are you going to do with your time?"

I had often thought of what I would say to him "if I could," but my answer turned out to be much milder than I had expected. I guess I was still inhibited from fully expressing my emotions by the fact that he *had* been my patient. I had to be satisfied with just explaining and describing how I felt, and as I was telling him how much his comments had always hurt me and how I had had to control my temper because of my professional obligation toward him, he kept interrupting me by insisting that he had been "kidding all along." But we all knew that he had not been kidding and that I was far angrier than I let myself appear. It was over, and we have not spoken to each other since.

What about friends who become patients? Some of these relationships go back to childhood or to college, and some are of a more recent vintage, but it is not at all unusual for a doctor to be asked to assume the medical care of someone with whom he has had a free-and-easy connection in the past.

It is, of course, easily understandable why a patient would choose a doctor who is already a friend. On paper at least, what could be more reassuring than being watched over by someone of whose goodwill you are already convinced? Isn't he going to go that extra mile for you when you really need him? Isn't the person who stays up with you until two in the morning, sipping cognac and discussing life, going to understand you and your emotional needs much better than a stranger?

It is also not hard to understand why a doctor is flattered when he realizes that his friends, in addition to liking him, have seen something else in him that has prompted them to put their lives in his hands. I can still remember the thrill, especially the first few times it happened to me, when a friend asked me to be his doctor. It was a great feeling, and especially because it suggested to me that the people who knew me in depth, faults and all, had that added confidence in my qualities that turned me from a friend into an all-around influence on their lives. When I was much younger, I had a need, out of insecurity, I am sure, to make an obvious impact on other people, so this dual role was very much up my emotional alley. Still, over the years, I sensed the warmth and esteem behind these requests, and my enthusiastic "Yes" in turn spoke for my gratitude.

Yet it comes as a shock to friends who become patients—and, to a certain extent, to patients who also become friends—that doctors cannot be "regular people" when they are on the job. Certainly my personal feelings for them do not change when they see me professionally, but in some ways I must seem to them to be a stranger. These patients have a fantasy that, though it is understandable, is still a fantasy, and that is that I am available to them twenty-four hours a day and that, for instance, inconvenient scheduling and having to tangle with my "overprotective" secretary will from now on be things of the past. And when I examine them, or suggest tests that might conceivably lead to unhappy diagnoses, I must seem vastly different to them from another me—let's say, the guy lying in front of the fire in his blue jeans after a day's skiing.

Certainly misunderstandings will arise. I had a dear old childhood friend whose teenage daughter once came in to see me with unexplained abdominal pain. In addition to routine laboraory studies, it is prudent to draw a pregnancy test in these situations, and it turned out to be negative. After the bill arrived from the laboratory, she was so angry at the very implication that she might be sexually active that she called me at home one evening during dinner and, after having told me that her father suggested she call, berated me for a full forty-five minutes before I finally suggested that we discuss the matter at another time. Another friend, one who had started out as a patient, once called me at six o'clock on a summer Saturday morning about the head lice she had found on her child. The reason for the unusual timing of the call? The family was leaving on vacation, and she wanted to be sure to get the medicine as soon as the pharmacy opened its doors several hours later. In these cases, which I, of course, give only as examples, the patients did not understand that even if the doctor is also a family friend, his time, his privacy, and his person must still be treated with respect. And why else do I still remember these little episodes after such a long time? I guess I have never given up on the idea, which is really a misunderstanding on my part, that, *especially* because the doctor is also a friend, he deserves consideration from the people who know him—and, presumably, love him—best.

This kind of experience is just a petty annoyance, and is not important enough to discourage a would-be friendship between patient and doctor. What is much more serious, though, is the emotional risk a doctor takes when he handles the critical illness of a friend or, worse yet, when a friend dies while he is under his care. As I have already said, the doctor's sense of objectivity and his ability to take a step back help him in taking good and clear-eyed care of the patient. But if a doctor is also a friend, then both he and the patient do not have the benefit of these safeguards. This does not mean that he cannot take good care of the patient, but he should be aware of the fact that he is under a handicap and that he has to make an allowance for this when making clinical decisions so they are not made on the basis of emotion rather than rational judgment.

One of the closest friends I ever had was Bob, a fellow resident in both hospitals where I took my training in internal medicine. When we graduated from the program, I immediately went into practice, but Bob decided to take a year off and go to Europe. His mother had died years before, and he rarely saw his brother, who lived in California. His father was thus Bob's only real family, so I was proud when Bob asked me to take over his father's medical care. But I was also a little frightened, and although I felt medically capable, I knew I would always be self-conscious about treating him. In addition, Bob was an excellent doctor, and I knew that somehow I would always feel forced to justify to him any medical decisions I made about his father. We had spent many, many hours during the years of our training talking about our feelings about medicine and especially about the heavy burden that comes with taking responsibility for another person's life. This was why it was not hard to describe to him what my concerns were. Yet when he began to go into his own feelings of guilt about leaving his father, who had already had one heart attack, while he set out to satisfy his longtime dream of living in Paris, and when he told me how reassured he would be if he knew his father was under my supervision, I had to agree to his request.

One Saturday evening (I also remember the date, the exact hour, the weather—in short, everything connected with that terrible night), Mac called me at home. His name was really Max, but possibly to widen his appeal as a clothing salesman, he liked to be called by a slightly less ethnic first name. There was no mistaking what he did for a living, though. Like many middle-aged men in the white-collar part of the garment business of that time, he wore tight-fitting suits and shirts with his monogram embroidered on the French cuffs, and, since men still wore hats in those days, he was never without a beautiful pearl-gray, snap-brim fedora. He was also the kind of man who insisted on paying for services rendered. Since it was obvious that I would not accept money from him, he had invited my wife and me to dinner on several occasions. He did not take us to standard places, but instead we went to old-speakeasies-turned restaurants that still, so many years after the repeal of prohibition, had no signs to identify them to the outside world. In these places, the steaks were great, the drinks had the thrill of the recently illicit about them, and Mac invariably stuffed some dollar bills into the stocking of the scantily dressed hatcheck girl when we left. Even though we were New Yorkers, my wife and I were real innocents, and those evenings gave us a taste of what life must have been like in the 1920s and 1930s. We always came home afterward feeling a little bit as if we had just spent the evening with one of those movie gangsters like George Raft.

But this time Mac was not calling to invite us to dinner. "I'm having bad chest pain, Pete," he said. "You better come right over!" I had, of course, been dreading what I was now hearing, since Bob had left for France a few weeks before. I felt a wave of panic in my own chest, and all I could think of at that moment was how I was going to explain it to Bob if his father died under my care. I knew that Mac always had nitroglycerin with him, so I instructed him to take two under his tongue right away. I asked him where he was, and when he gave me the address, it was an unfamiliar one. "I'm at a girl's house," he explained. It turned out that he was not far away, and I promised that it would take me only about ten minutes to reach him. It was obvious that he was having a heart attack and that he would have to be hospitalized immediately, so I asked him to have his friend call for an ambulance while I was on my way.

The initial panic had left me, but I was very worried as I drove up Park Avenue and then turned west on Eighty-sixth Street. This was going to be his second heart attack, and I was already preparing myself for the complications like shock or severe lung congestion that accompany a significantly damaged heart muscle. When I arrived at the address he had given me, a residential hotel at Eighty-sixth Street and Madison Avenue, I was disappointed to see that there was no ambulance waiting before the entrance, so I knew that it would still be a while before he could be taken to the hospital. In those days, doctors still carried bags in their cars, and I remember thinking how glad I was that I had replenished my supply of syringes and medications just the day before.

The lady who opened the door could certainly not be classified as a "girl." She appeared to be in her late forties or early fifties and wore her very red hair upswept à la Lucille Ball. She was wearing black toreador pants (they were the rage that year) with spiked-heel black pumps and a robin's-egg-blue low-cut sweater with a fur shawl collar, all of which she had put on in obvious anticipation of a long romantic evening with Mac. But tears had already made her makeup run, and I thought momentarily about how long it must have taken her to bring her face up to the standard of youthfulness suggested by her outfit. As she showed me into the living room, where Mac was lying propped up on the couch, she assured me that she had called for an ambulance. He was very pale and sweating profusely, his shirt was open (the gold cuff links were still in place, though), and his usually perfectly combed hair was in disarray. He was cradling the center of his chest with both hands, and as soon as he saw me he said, "Pete, I'm in terrible pain, you gotta do something," adding, "I've never had such bad pain, I think I'm gonna die!" With this, my vision of how it would be to have to tell Bob that his father had died came back full force, but my reflexes (which evidently had much more courage than the rest of me) took over, and I heard myself saying, "Mac, the hell you are, because I'd never find my way back to those dives that you took me to, and besides, I never even found out what they're called!"

The first thing to do was try to relieve the severe pain. After having taken his blood pressure, which was slightly lower than usual, I gave him an injection of a painkiller. While I waited for it to take effect, I examined him and was glad to see that he had no lung congestion, which would have made his condition even more serious. In the meantime, a policeman, usually the harbinger of the ambulance, had appeared and was making notes on the information provided by Ida, for that was the name of the "girl." Pain can in itself worsen matters, and when Mac's severe distress had not lessened within ten minutes of the first shot, I gave him a small additional dose of the same medication. Because of the unusually severe pain Mac was having, I began to wonder whether he did not really have an aortic dissection, a tearing of the main blood vessel in the chest, rather than a heart attack. It was plain that it was urgent that he get to a hospital as soon as possible, for diagnosis as well as for treatment, but just as I was about to ask the policeman to call again about the ambulance, we heard the sound of an approaching siren. Mac was still very pale, but alert enough to insist that I go with him in the ambulance to the hospital. As I was promising him that I would not let him out of my sight, the doorbell rang and the ambulance attendants, carrying a stretcher, came into the room. But in the very next moment, Mac let out a shriek of pain and, right after that, became unresponsive and stopped breathing. I could not hear a heartbeat, either, so it was obvious that he had had a cardiac arrest.

So far in this already very long evening, whenever I had a compulsive vision of what it would be like to tell Bob about what had happened to his father while I was supposed to be taking good care of him, it was really just an extension of the fearful fantasies I'd had since Bob entrusted him to me in the first place. But now, as I was drawing adrenaline up into a syringe connected to a long needle so I could inject the drug right into the heart in the hope of restarting the beat, and while the ambulance attendants were giving artificial respiration (effective resuscitation at that time was in its infancy, especially outside the hospital), I was no longer faced with a fantasy but with the full horror of the real situation. It was obvious that

Mac was dead, and after a few more minutes of various desperate maneuvers, we gave up.

Ida was kneeling next to the couch, holding one of Mac's hands and kissing it from time to time. I never did find out how close they were, but judging from the winks he gave us when Bob would kid him about his "harem," it was quite possible that there were a few more Idas spread around town. However, she cried as if she were the only one, or maybe she was representing all the possible others. The ambulance people were packing up their gear, and the policeman was phoning in his report, as I began to go through the transition from imagining the worst to experiencing the worst that could be imagined.

The death of a patient is always a wrenching experience for a doctor. But in this case, it was much, much worse. Because he was my best friend's father, and also because I was in a sense his guardian while Bob was away, I had been able to contribute very little objectivity to Mac's medical care while he was alive. But now that he was so shockingly dead, a whole range of irrational thoughts came over me. Was this just a bad dream, and was I going to wake up in the morning, as Bob must be doing now in Paris, to find out that Mac was in Ida's bed, safe and sound? However, the scene I was witnessing—though reminiscent, I suddenly thought, of the last moments of *La Traviata* and *La Bohème* combined, in which the irrevocable guarantee of death had conferred tragic roles on lover, doctor, and bystanders—was undeniably real.

What's more, I was frightened. Wouldn't Bob want to punish me with the weapon I could least defend against: namely, his scorn at my letting his father die? And that patron saint of sorrowful doctors, guilt, was right there as well. Where had I gone wrong? In reviewing what had happened during what seemed like every minute of the time between Mac's original phone call and his death, I could not find any glaring errors I had made. Yet that did not stop me from questioning tiny pieces of judgment—for instance, whether I should have run the red lights on my way to him in order to be there a few minutes earlier, or whether I should not have pushed for the ambulance to come quicker from the moment I arrived at Ida's apartment. I understood, of course, that a few minutes either way very rarely make the difference between a patient's life and death. But at that moment, I was even prepared to assume partial blame for this tragedy, anything rather than having to continue to feel the becalmed dread that had taken hold of me since I finally called a halt to our vain efforts to bring Mac back to life.

I stayed up all that night trying to find Bob. Fortunately, it took me a few hours to reach him, and by the time I did, I was much calmer. I had suffered so much already with the anticipation of how and what I would tell him of his father's death that the actual event was an anticlimax. Bob had never liked to show emotion, and even now he kept the conversation on a medical level, but I remember wishing he would show some grief so I could in turn vent my own feelings of sorrow at the way things had turned out. This standoff continued even after the funeral, and I never found out how Bob really felt about what had happened. Even though the reason for my feeling of guilt was not at all clear, I wanted him to release me from it, whatever its cause—in other words, to pardon me. We continued to be friends in the months that followed, but the unresolved issue of his father's death somehow always stood between us. I guess there is a statute of limitations even for guilt, though, because, happily, mine finally expired on its own after a year or two.

If I had it to do over again, would I ever combine friendship with doctoring? I am really not sure what the answer is. The experiences about which I have spoken here certainly show how complicated these double relationships can be. Yet, over the years, I have had memorable friendships with people who started out as patients, and on many occasions our professional relationship has strengthened the ties that I originally had with old friends. I realize that it would be helpful if I could give firm advice in this very murky area. But I cannot give a hard-and-fast judgment because even my own experience is mixed, so the whole issue is wrapped in the unpredictability of what is going to happen between people who want to be friends, and further complicated by the problematic nature of relations between doctors and patients. It's really too close to call, but if I had to choose, knowing what I do now, I would again take the chances I took over the years. I would not let my profession stand in the way of friendship.

At least the letters do not have to be changed. A VIP (Very Important Person) changes into a Very Important Patient almost automatically. Who should be considered a VIP? Is it old money, political power, or the presidency of a major corporation that magically transforms a "regular" patient into someone for whom schedules are changed, hard-to-get consultants are produced at the drop of a hat, and private hospital rooms are made available within minutes rather than the more usual days? The answer is yes in all these circumstances, but there are many others who qualify as well. In small towns, it may be the factory owner who hands out the most jobs or, for instance, the local sheriff. And in New York City, where the competition for status is as fierce as the one for money, being a big business-man may not be enough, so the would-be VIP may also have to be a major contributor to the hospital's building fund in order to qualify.

But what do doctors feel when they meet up with this exotic species? It would be insincere to claim that being picked out by a big shot to be his doctor is not a boost to the ego. Closeness to power is heady stuff, and it stimulates even the most jaded practitioner to new visions of glory. Yet there is a penalty attached to being only a star in the patient's firmament, rather than being in the usual situation, where the doctor is the sun around which all his patients cluster. To do our best work, we need a sense of independence from influences other than strictly medical ones. If the patient's importance makes the doctor too self-conscious or too sensitive to scrutiny, then he can't use his best judgment, and as a consequence the patient's care will suffer as well.

Despite their far-ranging contacts, VIPs do not necessarily go to the best doctors. As a matter of fact, they often go for brand names, physicians who are on lists titled "The 100 Best Doctors in ——," or they go to subspecialists recommended to them by other VIPs, when what they really need is a less famous but definitely competent family doctor.

Giving the same amount of attention and concern to every complaint, laboratory test, and physical finding is not only impractical but also subjects the patient to the undue worry that comes with excessive testing. What we call an experienced physician is someone who knows what is or is not important and who has the capacity to decide how seriously individual abnormalities have to be followed up. Doctors of VIPs, whose work is so constantly scrutinized, tend to do too much and do not let the reasonable and natural flow of diagnosis take place on its own.

I have always felt a lot of sympathy for the doctors of our presidents. When they are doing a good job, nobody pays much attention to them, as is the case with the rest of us as we deal with our less exalted patients. But when something is wrong, the judgment, good or bad, of the president's doctor is there for all to see. When a patient of mine called me with a story of a cough and low-grade fever for a couple of days, I usually handled it over the phone and advised the patient to stay in bed and to take cough medicine. But what if the president had the same complaints? Of course, I would see him and examine him (after all, we would both be working in the same place), but would I have the courage not to start him on antibiotics right away and not to do a chest x-ray (thinking all the while how it would make me look if he turned out to have a pneumonia that was not diagnosed early enough)?

Quite a few years ago, when I was still in training, I got a very good insight into the frenzy that can be generated around the serious illness of a major contributor to the hospital. Charles Gold, a major garment manufacturer, had been the chairman of the board of trustees for many years. He had been generous with both his time and his money, so wherever one turned, be it the emergency room, the operating room, or the house staff dormitories, there was a bronze plaque on the wall attesting to the endowment of the facility by either Charlie (as he was known to all—but, of course, not to his face) or by one of his relatives. He was a tall, gray-haired, handsome man in his seventies, with a blue flower invariably placed in his well-cut lapel, who could often be seen inspecting the hospital with the director and several administrators following at a respectful distance. Whenever he encountered one of our chiefs or senior attendings during one of these whirlwind tours, we interns and residents were always shocked to see how deferential they were to Charlie—pretty much to the same degree, come to think of it, that we were to them.

One day, the word came out that Charlie was to have a prostatectomy. He had been admitted to the grandest private room the hospital possessed, and the two semiprivate rooms on either side had been emptied of their occupants as well, so Charlie, by himself, had replaced nine patients! In the meantime, the chief of urology had been seen bringing a suitcase into one of the empty rooms and had been heard to say to one of the nurses that he was staying "for the duration." Through the grapevine, we also heard that Charlie's care throughout was to be managed only by chiefs—no intern or resident was to come into contact with him—and that even care of the IVs (a job that usually, of course, belonged to the lowest of the low, an intern like me) was to be under the direct control of the director of anesthesiology.

Over the next few days, everything that could go wrong did go wrong. He bled profusely from the area where the prostate had been removed, to the point where he had to be transfused with several units of blood. The worried little circle that stood together at least twice daily outside Charlie's room, and that included the chiefs of urology and anesthesiology and my boss, the chief of medicine, now included, because of the bleeding, the chief of hematology as well. After the hemorrhage had been controlled, Charlie spiked a high fever. The grapevine was not sure whether this was caused by a collapsed lung or by a wound infection, but by now the chief of pulmonary had joined the enlarging circle, which was meeting ever more frequently. In the meantime, Charlie's veins had been found to be terrible, and loud cries could be heard from his room when the head anesthesiologist tried, for the fourth or fifth time in a row, to thread a needle into a tiny vein, which invariably promptly burst. A vascular surgeon had to be called in, and he performed a little operation called a cutdown, which exposed a large vein into which a needle could be placed directly. In the meantime, some of the stitches had come out on their own, and the chief of surgery was consulted about what to do with the mutinous wound. Constipation, a common enough postoperative problem, worried the chiefs enough so that, when they could not agree on which laxative to give, the head of the gastroenterology section was called in for an opinion as well.

By the time Charlie finally went home, he had experienced far too much of what his hospital was capable of providing. The complications he had could have happened to anyone, but they are not at all unusual in patients whose doctors are trying just too hard. There is much to be said in favor of the "normal" system, under which doctors with a whole range of seniority and experience, from chiefs to interns, take care of the patient. What makes patients in general and VIPs in particular think that a nonsurgical chief who, though the possessor of large amounts of knowledge, has routinely delegated many clinical duties to his juniors for years can suddenly bounce back and be effective in, let's say, the evaluation and treatment of postoperative complications? Isn't it really better to be under the care of someone who, although not so senior, has the excellent reflexes that come with day-to-day, year-to-year experience in treating common clinical problems?

On paper, it makes sense to get the biggest doctor to take care of you. But in real life, the biggest is frequently not the best. Just because you have the home telephone number of the president of General Motors, does that mean he is the only one you will allow to fix your car?

There are some doctors I know who have any number of VIPs on their patient rosters. They walk around with x-ray folders emblazoned with names we usually see on theater marquees or on book jackets, and camera crews can be seen in front of their patients' hospital rooms. I was never one of them, although I admit that I was jealous when, for instance, my friend Abe was flown to Europe to consult on a famous movie producer who had had a stroke while on location, or when I was asked, in the lobby of the hospital, for directions to a colleague's office by someone I recognized as a Supreme Court justice recently named UN ambassador. On the one hand, we understand that a VIP is just another patient, though admittedly one who requires special handling, but on the other, we feel that being the doctor of a VIP somehow confers Very Important status on us as well. We doctors are highly competitive with each other, and in addition, we are all very vain. What better way is there to show our colleagues how important we are than to flaunt our famous patients before them like so many trophies?

In the early 1980s I had the opportunity of taking care of someone who, though not a hospital trustee or a politician or a famous actor or writer, was an irreplaceable natural resource. Arthur Rubinstein was at that time ninety-four years old and had come to New York from Paris in connection with the publication of the second volume of his autobiography. When his secretary called for an appointment I was surprised, because, as I have said, I did not belong to the group of VIP doctors, nor did I have any contacts in musical circles. It turned out that Rubinstein's daughter was an intern in another medical center, and that a former student of mine was her resident. She had asked him for the name of an internist for her father, and that is how I came to be called.

I had, of course, admired Rubinstein's playing for many years, and by coincidence was just reading the first volume of his autobiography. The book was enchanting, and I was very much under the spell of the charming stories he told about his long life. But to be able to meet him, to actually make human contact with him, had been extremely remote until just a few minutes before. Without even asking why he wanted to see me, I told my secretary to have him brought right over.

If I had expected to see the bubbly raconteur I had encountered in the book, I was very wrong. Instead, I saw a silent, pale, very old little man wearing a voluminous coat, scarf, and hat (it was May) sitting immobile in a wheelchair. With him was an attractive Englishwoman in her mid-thirties who was his secretary-companion and who asked me to call her Annabel. He was obviously quite deaf, but after Annabel had introduced me, not speaking too loudly but enunciating each word very clearly, he did open his eyes and say, *"Bonjour."* Rubinstein's companion gave a very clear history. He had two chief problems. One was that he had severe low back pain, which was being treated with pain medication and which had been diagnosed as sciatica by a doctor at the American Hospital in Paris. The other was that he had to get up a dozen times a night to urinate and that he had a constant urge to void during the day as well. When I asked Annabel how long the back pain had been going on, she told me that it had just been for the past several months.

The patient was obviously in no shape to undergo a complete physical examination, so I invoked what is known in medicine as Sutton's law. Willie Sutton was a famous bank robber, and not a scientist or clinician, but the reason he has ended up in our special vocabulary is that, when asked why he specifically robbed banks, he replied, "Because that's where the money is!" As far as I was concerned, when a ninety-four-year-old man has had a recent onset of back pain, it is much less likely to be sciatica than a cancer of the prostate with spread to bone. I therefore went right for the money—the prostate, in this case—and found what I expected, a large, hard lump.

When Annabel rolled the patient into my consultation room a few minutes later, I quickly realized that he was completely alert and that, if I imitated the way she spoke to him, he understood everything I told him. What's more, even though he had very poor eyesight, I was astonished to hear him pick out the name of the artist (Chagall) responsible for the original of the Metropolitan Opera poster advertising *The Magic Flute* that was hanging on the far wall of the office. His lethargy had probably been caused by too large a dose of the pain medication (old people are notoriously sensitive to sedation and usually require smaller doses than younger people), but now that that effect was wearing off, and if Annabel's example was followed as far as his hearing was concerned, Arthur Rubinstein could clearly be seen to be intellectually entirely intact! So much for the unfortunate tendency all of us have to diagnose senility far too quickly rather than first considering drug effect or sensory deprivation as a cause for what only *looks* like intellectual deterioration in old people.

I arranged for immediate hospitalization (the admitting office clerk must have been a music lover—no questions asked), and over the next several days, the CAT scans, bone scans, and blood tests all confirmed my diagnosis. On a much smaller dose of the pain medication, Arthur (that's what he invited me to call him, with the accent on the last syllable, French style) perked up remarkably. He had accepted the news calmly, and agreed to undergo surgery for both palliation of his cancer and relief of his urinary tract obstruction. Although, despite my admiration for him, I was all business at the beginning of our relationship, I now found it difficult to make even the smallest decisions about him. These ranged from the choice of urologic surgeon (should it be the chief, notoriously uncommunicative with patient and doctor, or should it be one [but which one?] of the more junior but still very capable attendings in the department?) to whether or not I should depend on the luck of the draw as far as an anesthesiologist was concerned (or should I ask for one of the elite, the ones who worked with the cardiac surgeons?). The medical workup I had instituted showed that his heart and lungs were in remarkably good order, but I still feared some unforeseen event during or immediately after surgery that could kill this unique man.

My hospital visits were notoriously short, and though I was thorough and didn't just wave from the door, they were still short. Over the years, I should not have been so contemptuous of the "celebrity doctors" who were known to spend large chunks of time with their Very Important Patients, because I found myself doing the same thing. Now that he knew that something definitive was to be done for him, whatever the diagnosis, Rubinstein was very cheerful, and each time I saw him, he wore a beautiful silk dressing gown with a matching pocket handkerchief, his feet encased in embroidered velvet slippers, and he smelled of an unfamiliar cologne, which he said was a special fragrance made for him by Chanel. He was very talkative and so witty that his book, which I had found to be so extraordinary, had to be rated a distant second behind his actual presence.

It was my custom to see my hospital patients once a day, and twice if they were seriously ill. I found myself seeing Arthur three or four times a day and staying about half an hour each time. The frequent visits were not necessary medically—as a matter of fact, everything had finally been arranged and we were just waiting for operating time—but I was so fascinated by him, and had begun to like him so much, that I felt physically drawn to see him as often as I could. Yet he was unlike any VIP I had ever heard of. He made no demands, went along with all my suggestions, and left the choice of doctors entirely up to me. As a matter of fact, when I tried to give him a choice (of surgeons, let's say), he would invariably reply, "You are my Doktor Leben, I trust you!" I had heard this term *Doktor Leben* before, because that is what my father's Orthodox Jewish patients had called him when he was still practicing in Austria. *Leben* means "life," but when it is appended to the term *Doktor* it is an endearment that suggests another, more familiar, Jewish phrase: "You should live and be well!"

I admit it, I was hooked. Solid citizens, when they fall from grace, can be outrageous in their behavior. I had certainly never been intrusive with my patients, and I usually tended to hold back, at least for a while, when personal contact with a patient was in the offing. But in Rubinstein's case, it was a combination of a tremendous desire to pull him out of his illness even at this advanced stage of his life and my attraction to someone who was a link, and an infinitely attractive link at that, with a world of music and of good living that is only legendary for people of my generation, which made me pull out all the stops in the admittedly oversolicitous attention I gave him.

On the day of his operation, I woke up very early. He was the first case, and I wanted to be sure to check him one more time before he went to the operating room. When I arrived, Annabel, who slept on a cot in his room, was already up, but our star patient was sleeping peacefully. Annabel and I spoke in the nervous, fitful way that people do when something with unknown consequences is about to befall them. When Arthur woke up, though, he immediately made us laugh as he imitated Vladimir Horowitz, who had been the principal player in the dream from which he had just awakened.

The anesthesiologists are justifiably called the internists of the operating room. A generic internist like myself therefore has very little reason to attend operations, and actually has no authority at all once his patient crosses the threshold of the operating suite. Yet in Rubinstein's case, because of his advanced age and my fears for his safety, I emphatically told the surgeon, anesthesiologist, and anyone else who would listen that I would be nearby throughout the procedure and that I should be notified immediately if anything went wrong. For the next two hours, I fidgeted about, going in and out of the operating room every few minutes and generally probably acting and definitely feeling like an anxious relative. Although patients very rarely die during surgery, operations have always made me nervous. The combination of forcibly putting a patient to sleep together with cutting deep into his body, although admittedly necessary and frequently life-saving, does have a violent aspect to it that does not mesh well with certain temperaments—like mine, for example. So I was very anxious all the while that Arthur was lying there unconscious with a breathing tube down his throat. But the monitor showed a normal rhythm, the blood gases were excellent, and the surgeon was whistling (usually an optimistic sign, except in those few cases where they whistle only when they are terrified), so I was reassured to some degree that Arthur was going to come out of all this alive.

It has always seemed to me that good basic health is necessary if a patient is going to live into his nineties. Arthur's uncomplicated progress postoperatively supported this suspicion of mine, and he was discharged from the hospital five days after the surgery. My compulsive watch over him did not stop, of course, and I continued to see him at home daily and spoke another two to three times a day on the telephone to Annabel.

Before the operation, we had decided that we would have a "victory lunch," my treat, when Arthur was feeling better. Not only that, but we had agreed that he would not leave New York before he could walk into the plane, in contrast to his arrival, when he had had to be taken off in a wheelchair.

I had made a reservation for late in the lunch hour at one of my favorite restaurants, beautifully situated on Park Avenue in the Fifties. Its main entrance, coatroom, and rest rooms are situated on the ground floor. A floating stairway ends at the bar and then a lofty passageway, presided over by a magnificent, huge tapestry, leads to a dining room that has a shimmering marble pool as its centerpiece. Happily, the upper part of the restaurant has an emergency exit onto Park Avenue, so Annabel could walk Arthur in from street level, thus avoiding the stairs.

Arthur looked splendid in a beautifully cut double-breasted blue suit, striped shirt, and a pearl stickpin in his light blue silk tie. I began with a champagne toast to his recovery, and he then took over with a toast to Doktor Leben, then one to the "faithful" Annabel, then one to the "beautiful" Adrienne (my wife). At my request, he imitated Horowitz again, and then he was off and running with several other imitations, among them

195

Toscanini and Stokowski. By this time it was about two-thirty, and the restaurant was beginning to empty, but we had not even gotten to the main course yet. At this point, he leaned over to me and whispered, "Doktor Leben, where can one make *pipi?*" I immediately saw the full horror of the situation. The men's room was below, we were up here, and he certainly could not navigate the stairs. The operation had drastically cut down on the number of times he had to urinate, but I really should have thought of this contingency.

I have always been a believer in inviting people only to restaurants I know well. If the host is as ignorant as the guests of the strengths and weaknesses of the kitchen or of the wine list, then he is really inept. In this case, though, I was very glad that I knew the restaurant as well as I did, and it had nothing to do with the food or wine. It had to do, rather, with a small coatroom located in the passageway between the bar and the dining room in which we were sitting. Medicine, of course, is all about problem solving, as well as the utilization of whatever means are necessary to relieve the patient's distress. Therefore I had no qualms about what I was going to do. I asked Arthur to get up and walked him to the little coatroom, which was really a counter with a small closet in the back, and which was unattended. I asked him to wait for me there and went on to the bar. I then asked the bartender on duty, in a very matter-of-fact way, to give me a wine carafe. I must have looked very authoritative because he gave me one without question, and I carried it back to the coatroom. I asked Arthur to step into the little closet with the carafe while I stood guard outside. It was obvious that the urologist had made a large channel in Arthur's prostate, because it took him only about two minutes to fill up half the carafe, which he then handed back to me. My deep-seated reflexes stayed with me even in this outlandish situation, because I remember looking at the urine in the carafe and admiring its clarity and lack of obvious pus or blood. The immediate question, however, was what to do with the half-full carafe. I couldn't take it back to the bartender, because that would have really been unseemly. I could not take it downstairs to empty it, because I had nothing to wrap it in. I certainly could not take it back to the table, so I had only one choice. I placed it on the floor of the little closet, hoping for the forgiveness of the perplexed maintenance crew that was bound to find it sooner or later. Arthur and I then innocently walked back to our table, looking for all the world, except that we were laughing so hard, as if I had just shown him, in some detail, the beautiful tapestry that was such a trademark of the restaurant.

Several weeks later, Arthur did walk into the Air France plane to Paris under his own power. I saw him once more before he died, after he had broken his hip, when Annabel called me to come over and see him "just to make sure." He has been dead for more than ten years, but he is not at all forgotten. His records, which are now on CDs, are very popular, and a new biography is going to be coming out. I said before that I was sometimes jealous of the "VIP doctors," but that was before I met Arthur. Being his "Doktor Leben" was a once-in-a-lifetime experience and worth waiting for until the third decade of my practice. I was usually extroverted and demonstrative with my patients, and yet I was also circumspect and watchful of the formalities in the relations between patients and doctors. This once I deviated knowingly from the "professional manner" that is so necessary for us to maintain, and I replaced it with open admiration tinged with wistfulness that I had met him so very late in his life. In short, I "lost my cool" completely, and I will always be glad that I did.

10

Malpractice and Mispractice

MALPRACTICE IS AN issue that has been talked to death. Health advocates, patients, doctors, and doctors' organizations all have strong opinions on the subject, even though many people do not have a clear idea at all of what it is. In recent years, doctors have been able to breathe a little easier as far as suits are concerned. What we have been saying for years, that the high premiums we pay have to be passed on to the patient in some way and that the "defensive medicine" some of us have been pushed into costs the country a fortune, seems to have finally made an impression. The rules are being changed by some states, and the awards seem to be getting smaller, so it appears that the malpractice "crisis" is probably going to be over one of these days.

What is not going to be over for a long time, though, is how we doctors feel about what we have gone through. Insurance companies, state governments, medical organizations, and the judicial system that used to hand out huge awards can afford to declare an armistice in this particular war between patients and doctors. But what happens to the bad feeling and distrust between those who were just foot soldiers in the battle? How are the patients going to express the anger and resentment they still feel so strongly toward us if they cannot, at least, have their feelings soothed by money? And how should we feel toward those who, until it seems only yesterday, had the right to mug us in broad daylight while we were in the middle of doing our jobs? Should we now drop our guard and erase from our memories the dry throat that came with the serving of the subpoena, the restless nights, and the fear of financial ruin when we realized that the claim was for several million dollars more than the face value of our policies?

What's more, how can I get rid of even that slight feeling of distrust I feel toward my patients, including those who are very unlikely to sue? Can I go "all out" for my patients if I am afraid of them at the same time? If I give in to my fears, isn't every patient I see the potential destroyer of my life? Since large amounts of money are at stake, can't any action or lack of action on my part be interpreted as malpractice if things go badly, even though I am not at fault?

Of course, things are not usually as bad as all that, and I don't want to give the impression that I thought of nothing else but the threat of a malpractice suit day and night. Whether we are a little afraid of our patients or not, their health is still our biggest worry. Besides, the insurance companies and Medicare have seen to it that our blood pressures rise every day when the mail is delivered, so fears of being sued have had to stand in line and wait their turn to get our attention.

The whole idea of doctors being held accountable for malpractice is a worthwhile one. Yet it has gotten a bad name because it cannot separate itself from the widespread impression that there is some stable exchange rate between money and suffering. Doctors who do bad things to patients, out of ignorance or negligence, *should* be weeded out. Isn't it just more evidence of the cowardly "no fault" quality of our society that an insurance company pays a patient for that favorite, pain and suffering, while the doctor who is responsible is often allowed to go on, no smarter than before? Where is the moral indignation, the anger, that the patient who has had the wrong leg cut off, or the one who is allowed to go into diabetic coma despite obvious symptoms of diabetes, is supposed to feel? Is money finally really supposed to take care of everything? Is this the way to see to it that patients don't get victimized generation after generation?

Most cases of malpractice are very obvious, and patients suffer and die because of some outrageous act on the part of a doctor. It does not take some close decision by a jury, after a clever reconstruction of the case by the plaintiff's lawyer, to convince us that malpractice has actually taken place. I have been a member of a state medical malpractice mediation panel, and I have done expert review of cases for lawyers. The lawyer and the judge who were the other members of the panel and I always were unanimous in our decision—which almost always was in the plaintiff's favor, by the way. What's more, after my expert reviews, I have often recommended that the insurance company settle with the plaintiff, since I felt that he was justified in his accusations and that the doctor had a very poor case.

Ruth Frank was the mother of not one, but two, child psychiatrists. She was a quiet, unassuming lady who had the type of diabetes that could have been easily controlled if she had only been able to limit her food intake. As it was, she was quite obese, and I threatened her frequently with the prospect of having to take insulin. Yet I always relented at the last minute when she promised, "You'll see how much weight I've lost next time you see me." She lived fairly far away, in New Jersey, but still she managed to see me every few weeks. On my recommendation, she was also seeing a local doctor so she would have someone to see in case of emergency, and I always made sure that he was fully informed of what my findings were.

I knew her sons well. The older one, Ted, had spent part of his internship under my supervision, and Jack, the younger one, had become my patient along with Marilyn, his wife. Their father, Aaron, had also been my patient until his death. So the Franks and I had an old, and close, relationship.

One day, Ted called me and told me that his mother had died that morning. I was, as usual, shocked by the "unexpected" death of a patient of mine, and especially because Ruth and her family were very dear to me. Ted seemed calm—he was not crying as far as I could tell—and so it seemed safe to ask him what had happened. I immediately remembered that she and I had spoken a few days before, when she had called me with symptoms typical of a cold but with no fever. I had asked her to call back if she did not get better within several days but had not heard from her since. Her upper respiratory symptoms went away quickly, Ted said. Yet, two days before, she mentioned to him, during their regular daily telephone conversation, that she was suddenly belching a lot and feeling some pressure in her lower chest as well.

He was a psychiatrist, of course, but I was glad to see that he had not forgotten everything he had learned as a medical intern. He told me that he had immediately asked his mother to call the local doctor and to see him that day. When he checked with her later on, she reported to him that the doctor had told her, over the telephone, that her symptoms were probably due to a lingering cold and that it did not sound to him as if she needed to be seen as an emergency. In the meantime, her chest pressure had lessened, but Ted was concerned enough to try to call the doctor. He could not be located by his answering service, though, so Ted never got a return call from him. By eleven o'clock at night, he tried to convince his mother to go to the local emergency room so she could have an electrocardiogram. By that time her symptoms had almost gone, and she refused, but she promised him that she would call me in the morning. Her sister-in-law, another widow, who lived with her, found her dead in bed that same night, and that was the end of the story.

Ted sounded more and more furious as he was telling me all this, and I could easily understand why. As I was listening, I became agitated myself, because it sounded to me as if Ruth had begun to have a heart attack at the time her new symptoms started, the day before. An obese, elderly, inactive, diabetic woman is a real setup for coronary artery disease, and chest pressure and belching, especially if they are new symptoms, which they were for her, should have alerted her doctor to the possibility of a heart attack. There was no question in my mind that he should have seen her as an emergency and that he should have put her in the hospital for observation, whether the first electrocardiogram showed anything abnormal or not.

Ted and his brother, Jack, came to see me a few weeks later. They wanted to thank me for taking care of their mother all those years, but the real reason for their visit was to discuss the malpractice suit they were filing against their mother's local doctor.

Patients, or their surviving relatives, are not likely to talk to one doctor about suing another one, probably because they feel that they are not going to get an honest opinion. No matter how much we try to rid them of the notion, they probably still believe, deep down, that we cover up for each other, so how can they expect the truth under these circumstances?

The Frank brothers were both doctors, so they understood as well as I did that the "cover-up" is almost always a complete myth. They were also different in another way, though, from the usual plaintiffs, and that was that they were suing for only $1 in damages! In other words, the case was going to have to go to trial, since they were obviously not going to settle for a lesser amount out of court.

From what I had heard, they seemed to have a strong case. What's more, since they were not trying to make money on their mother's misfortune, their motive seemed pure, and that was to draw attention to the negligent way in which the doctor had taken care of her. I could only agree with what they were doing. Of course, there was always the chance that the story was somehow "off," that the doctor was being accused falsely because Ruth had misunderstood something he said to her, and that she had then repeated only what she thought she heard when she spoke later to her son. Yet she had been an alert woman, and her son, a psychiatrist, was trained to listen carefully to what was told to him. What's more, she was not seen by the doctor the day before her death, and her son could not reach him despite many attempts, so it sounded, at least, as if the doctor was at fault. In all fairness, I could only hope that, if the doctor was unfairly accused, the examination before the trial and the trial itself would bring that out, but I felt that Ruth's sons had a good reason for going ahead with what they were planning, and I told them so.

It turned out that they won their $1, which did not cover their legal fees, which, at least in this case, were not covered by the usual contingency arrangement. Their winning the case did not lessen their grief, I am sure, and they lost money rather than making it. I can only hope that the doctor who was found guilty understood the point they were making, which had nothing to do with financial rewards for suffering and everything to do with conscientious caring for the lives of other people's mothers.

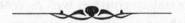

Giving general anesthesia to a patient known to have an overactive thyroid, and in the process causing a life-threatening condition known as thyroid storm; not properly diagnosing toxemia, thus not preventing seizures in a pregnant patient; diagnosing a "cold" without doing a chest x-ray in a patient with shortness of breath and high fever who turns out to have severe pneumonia; all these and, unfortunately, many others, are examples of *unacceptably bad* medicine. No decent doctor would defend this kind of negligence and incompetence, nor would he use these examples to try to show how unjustly we are often treated in matters of supposed malpractice.

How about the many other cases, then, the ones that are not at all obvious, many of which turn out to have no merit? I do not mean to say that there are not some perfectly justified suits that are based on more subtle evidence of malpractice. Yet it seems to me that the farther away we get from unquestionably bad care rendered by a doctor, the more we end up in a never-never land where hard evidence is replaced by innuendo and suggestion based on very little, if any, evidence that something wrong has been done to the patient.

This is the most dangerous area for decent doctors. An unpredictable illness, spotty cooperation on the part of the patient, unexpected responses to medications; all these can suddenly place the doctor in a very exposed and vulnerable position. It does not have to be for long, and he may recoup very quickly, but if that brief time is captured, as if on a freeze-frame in a video-tape, and it is cleverly produced as evidence, then *every one of us*, working on *any of the cases* that we have ever been involved in, could at some time in his life be accused guilty of malpractice.

There should be very little question about the motives of patients who have been the victims of obvious malpractice. They deserve their day in court as well as whatever else it takes to make it up to them for their misfortune. What about the marginal cases, though, the ones where the patient or his family goes to a lawyer to find out whether they have a "good case" or not? What is their main motive? I am not one of those who are convinced that money is at the root of all suits. Very few plaintiffs will go as far as asking for only $1 in damages, as the Frank brothers did, but I think that for many of them anger at the doctor comes first, only to be followed by the perfectly pleasant prospect of getting some money as well.

Why the anger? Doctors are well known to antagonize

patients with their bad behavior, and what better way is there to get back at them than with at least the nuisance value of a suit? Yet I do not think that pure revenge for these transgressions is a frequent motive, either; it is, rather, a misunderstanding of *what is not* malpractice that is often at the bottom of the problem.

Every time something unexpected happens to the patient, it is not malpractice! The idea of accident is very hard to accept when we are dealing with illness, although chance is accepted as the cause of auto or plane crashes, for example. Yet the public cannot get itself to go along with the notion that random, uncontrollable events can happen even though the patient is under the supervision of a doctor. This disbelief comes from a fantasy, and that is that the doctor is the middleman between fate and the human race. When something unexpected happens, isn't it then more practical to blame the always available middleman rather than slippery fate?

In medicine, when something goes wrong unexpectedly, it is most often chance that is to blame. The deadly allergic reaction to medication in a patient with no history of allergy, the postoperative heart attack in a patient with no previous history of heart disease—these complications, and others like them, belong to what I call my "torpedo scenario." The night is dark, and my patient and I are on a ship. All possible precautions have been taken against an attack by enemy submarines, which are known to be in the area. Yet one of them sends a torpedo our way, and it hits our ship. My patient is either injured or killed by the explosion, while I remain unhurt.

Was it malpractice on my part that was responsible for the harm to my patient? No, it wasn't. It would have been if I had not seen to it that all state-of-the-art safeguards against submarines were being taken, or if I had sent the patient on this dangerous trip by himself, without my supervision and support. As it was, I did my very best to protect him, but even the very best I have to offer does not control chance.

Understandably, patients find it very hard to believe us when we say (as we have always said, by the way) that, despite our best efforts, with all our theorizing, with all the use of our considerable experience, with all our studying, and with all our worrying, we can still not be right, or make accurate predictions, 100 percent of the time. In other words, we are not nearly as perfect as you want us to be, and what's more, we never will be. Beyond that, it is religion, fate, metaphysics, or whatever you want to call it; but it is no longer medicine practiced by other, fallible, human beings.

About fifteen years ago, I was asked to consult on an elderly lady who was hospitalized on the dermatology unit. She was extremely fat, and although her skin condition was improving, she had fever and abdominal pain, which led to my being asked to see her. She obviously had acute diverticulitis, an inflammation of little sacs that pop out of the colon, a condition that can be very serious if it is not treated promptly and thoroughly. I moved her that same day to the surgical floor, where she was treated for several weeks with antibiotics and IV fluids. Meanwhile, in order to put her colon to rest, she received nothing by mouth, and after a while she began to improve.

Mrs. Simone weighed maybe three hundred pounds, even after three weeks without solid food, yet her husband was half her size. He was always there when I came to visit, and never failed to ask me about her condition after I had finished examining her. They seemed very close. I knew that they were childless, and sometimes I would surprise them holding hands while they were watching television. She clearly needed to have the piece of colon that was inflamed removed; the CAT scan showed so much disease that it was risky to leave it in place. On the other hand, she was a terrible surgical risk because of her obesity. The surgeon and I talked over all the possibilities with the Simones, and we all finally agreed that it was safer to operate then, with the inflammation under control, than at some time in the future when the diverticulitis might be much worse.

It is not at all unusual to be pleasantly surprised by a patient's postoperative course. We had expected lung complications, wound infections, and the like, but she "sailed through," as we like to say, and a week after the operation we were able to transfer her to the convalescent unit. Mr. Simone appeared overjoyed. Relief at his wife's obvious improvement had somehow filled out his thin little frame, and even though they still looked like a very unlikely pair, it was possible, with a little bit of imagination, to see them as a couple.

After she had been in the cooperative care unit, our convalescent facility, for a few days, she complained one morning of a vague pain in her upper abdomen. At the same time I noticed that she was trembling. Her temperature was normal, yet she looked pale, so it seemed to me that something was again going on. An obese lady with upper abdominal pain has gallbladder trouble until proven otherwise, but when we reviewed her previous CAT scans, no stones were seen in the region of the gallbladder. When I saw her again, a few hours later, she was no longer trembling; she was now having shaking chills, and her temperature was 102 degrees. By the next morning, despite large amounts of antibiotics and fluids, she was worse, and it was obvious that she had to be operated on again. With her fever, and after a sleepless night, Mrs. Simone was listless, and when I started to talk to her about what needed to be done, she told me, with a wave of her hand, "Speak to Joe. He's in charge!"

It is always difficult to justify a second operation during the same hospitalization. When emergency surgery needs to be done on someone who is just convalescing from another operation, the doctors on the case have some explaining to do. I admitted to Joe right off the bat that we were not sure what was going on. The only thing we did know, I told him, was that she would die if we did not remove whatever was causing the new infection in her belly. A CAT scan done a few hours before had not shown any new diverticulitis, so it seemed possible that she had an inflamed gallbladder without the customary stones, a condition sometimes seen after abdominal surgery, especially after a long time of NPO (nothing by mouth). Joe had been looking at me suspiciously all morning, and now he said, "Hey, Doc, you guys wouldn't be pulling the wool over my eyes, would you? I mean, how do I know the first surgery wasn't screwed up and the trouble now is from that?"

I was not surprised by what he said. I had expected him to wonder whether he was being told the truth, so I told him what the most recent CAT scan had shown, that the problem did not seem to have anything to do with diverticulitis and that we thought the gallbladder was most likely to blame for the worsening of his wife's condition. He listened to me very carefully and looked maybe a little less on his guard when I finished, although I could tell that the whole story still did not make a lot of sense to him. Yet he signed the consent for surgery after I reassured him that his wife's medical condition, as far as I could tell after examining her and checking her chest x-ray and electrocardiogram, seemed to be unchanged from the past.

To no one's surprise, she had a very inflamed gallbladder without stones, which was removed. She went through the operation without difficulty, and ultimately she was transferred from the recovery room to the surgical ICU. The first night she was there, she suddenly went into shock; the electrocardiograms that were done showed a rapidly developing heart attack, and by the time I got to the hospital she had had a cardiac arrest and could not be resuscitated.

I never saw Joe after she died. I searched for him that day and tried to call him a few times after that, but I never got to speak to him. A few days later, I went to the surgical conference, where all deaths and complications are discussed. The chief was known for his brutally frank investigations, and he had everyone on the staff who was at all connected with Mrs. Simone's case on the carpet for more than an hour. Yet no matter how hard he tried, he could not find anything wrong with the way she had been handled by them. After her death, I had reviewed all her tests and cardiograms again. After all, I had cleared her for surgery; had I missed something on the EKG, or was there a laboratory test that was trying to tell me something that I ignored?

Though guilt-prone as I always have been, I could find nothing wrong with my handling of the situation, either. Would I have handled her differently if I had had another shot at her? No, she needed both operations; she was watched very carefully by the surgeons and me, and the heart attack that killed her was due to many things: two operations under general anesthesia (one soon after the other), obesity, and advanced age, all having their effect on a coronary artery that was very probably already narrowed to begin with.

I tell this story in such detail not to try to justify what we did but, rather, because this is the kind of case that is typically presented to a malpractice lawyer. The result was bad, the lady needed two operations; somebody must have done something wrong! Later on, all of us connected with the Simone case—the surgeons, the anesthesiologist, and I—were notified that we were being sued for malpractice. But before that, Joe had begun to call the surgeons' office, and mine as well, and although he never asked to speak to any of us personally, he left us some very disquieting messages. "Tell the doctor he killed my wife and my life the same day" was one, while another addressed itself to our futures: "I wish him a long life so he has plenty of time to feel all alone, like me!"

Joe always made a good impression on me, and I liked the way he had paid so much attention to his wife during her illness. The combination of the messages and the suit suggested to me that he was so angry that his wife had died, and that he missed her so much, that he had to pin her death on somebody. The money he might possibly be awarded, *if* he won the suit, seemed to me to be of lesser importance to him, and I liked him for that.

A certain number of malpractice suits, though, do not seem to have any motive other than to make money. There is the smell of the lottery about them, and the procedure goes something like this:

Step 1—You go to the doctor and pay his fee. (THE BET.)

Step 2—Something goes wrong, and you would like to think it's the doctor's fault, so you file suit. (THE WHEEL SPINS.)

Step 3—A jury finds in your favor. (YOUR NUMBER COMES UP—THE PAYOFF!)

Just as there are some relatives like the Franks, who did not want money in return for their mother's life, and Joe Simone, who sued out of grief, there are, predictably, some people who see a financial bonanza in their dealings with the doctor. They are the patients who are most likely to make us miserable, because for them malpractice is purely a business proposition. The average patient or relative is sometimes more, sometimes less, alert as far as possible malpractice is concerned. But the patient whose *purpose* it is to make money is actively looking for reasons to sue. We doctors are used to dealing occasionally with dissatisfied, angry, and even hostile patients, some of them having a perfectly reasonable beef, by the way. If they turn out to sue, we are emotionally prepared for it, because patients' complaints are still within our general experience in practicing medicine. Yet how do you get used to being held up? How do we know which of our patients considers us the instrument of his financial salvation? These are the ones who blindside us, those we cannot protect ourselves against, and those who are the most dangerous for our peace of mind. In addition, we are also on very weak ground, because now it is business—making money—that is at stake and not medicine, which at least we know something about. Since almost any action of ours can be picked out and used to make a case where there really is none, it turns out that we have to defend ourselves on a very broad front. In other words, instead of focusing all our energies on making our patients better, we spend far too much of our time and efforts in protecting ourselves against them; and that is the real tragedy of our malpractice system.

It is one thing to just be afraid of being sued for malpractice and quite another to be an actual defendant. The Bill of Particulars—the actual complaint or accusation—usually includes some pretty strong language. Words like *unprofessional, unfaithful, unskilled, careless, negligent,* and *reckless* are thrown about in the document, words you thought would never be tied not only to your name but also to the "Doctor" in front of it. Of course, whatever the Bill of Particulars says, that does not mean that you are guilty, but it is still a shock to even be accused of behavior you spent your entire professional life avoiding. What's more, just being accused takes its toll on you. Especially because the legal process is so slow, the doctor has a lot of time to worry about what is going to happen. Are they going to sue for more than the amount I am covered for, to force me into pushing my insurance company to settle rather than taking the chance of having to pay the difference myself? Even though the other defendants and I have talked it over many times and still feel that we acted correctly throughout, won't the jury have more sympathy for the grief-stricken little widower than for us seemingly powerful and rich doctors?

The lawyers assigned to us by the insurance company were reassuring. After a careful look at Mrs. Simone's hospital record, they could see nothing that could point a finger at us as far as bad practice was concerned. I was a little reassured, but since I have spent so many years cautioning patients that doctors cannot guarantee results, I knew very well that lawyers work under the same handicap. I understood that those terrible words in the Bill of Particulars were meant to make a point, for legal reasons, but I could not help being insulted by them. When I awoke at night, which was often in those days, I alternated between being frightened of the outcome of the case and being angry about the accusations. The others, the surgeons and the anesthesiologist, had been sued many times, par for the course for those specialties, and they advised me to relax. But it was my first time, and I just could not take it in stride as they did.

Joe had continued to call occasionally, even after the suit had been started. At the beginning, after his wife died, he had called almost every week, but by now it was once every month or six weeks, although what he said was pretty much unchanged from before. One day, though, our lawyer called, and at first I thought he wanted to discuss the upcoming EBT (Examination Before Trial). Instead, he told me that the suit had been dropped! He did not seem to want to go into the possible reasons for the sudden turnaround, so I thanked him for his help and hung up the phone.

I think I was right about Joe all along. He had always seemed like a reasonable man before, and I thought it was very possible that he had become reasonable again, many months after his wife's death. I was, of course, very grateful to be off the hook, but strangely enough, I was also indebted to Joe. He must have had a good enough case (as far as making money, and not necessarily as far as our guilt was concerned), otherwise a lawyer, who works on contingency, would not have taken it on. Yet he dropped the case. Didn't the cancellation of the suit mean the same thing as the lessening of the phone calls, an end to his mourning? That is my favorite explanation. What it says is that Joe not only took pity on us in stopping the suit when he began to realize that we were not at fault, but that he also took pity on himself and made a decision to continue with his life.

It is bad enough that we oftentimes cannot agree on whether or not malpractice has occurred, but even worse that we can't agree on what the word really means. A decision by a jury, either way, does not really make us much wiser; all it tells us is that the jurors had the impression, based on what was presented to them, that it did or did not happen. Yet although things are already so confusing, we need to add another word that is probably going to confuse us even more, but it covers a lot of unclear situations that come up between doctors and patients.

If *malpractice* means "bad practice," then what does the new word, *mispractice*, mean? It means that an error, a mistake, has been made in taking care of a patient, one that is usually easily corrected and does not cause any long-lasting ill effects. From what I have seen, there is, fortunately, much much more mispractice than malpractice, and frequently the patient is not even aware of it.

An elderly patient of mine, for instance, was found to have an abnormally low blood pressure while she was in the recovery room after breast surgery. Her electrocardiogram was unchanged, and there was no suggestion of internal bleeding, so the surgical residents decided to increase her IV fluids, thinking that dehydration might have caused her blood pressure to drop. Yet the more fluids she got, the lower her blood pressure became. It turned out that nobody had checked when the patient had urinated last, and she had a large amount of urine in her bladder. A stomach swollen with air, or a bladder swollen with urine, is well known to drop the blood pressure. When the urine was removed with a catheter, her pressure came right back to normal. What had happened was an error in judgment. There was no neglect or carelessness on the part of the residents taking care of her, just a delay in making the right diagnosis.

This is what happened to my son, a healthy twenty-five-year-old living in a big midwestern city. He fell ill with a high fever and symptoms of a cold. We were in frequent touch by telephone, and for the first two days I was not really concerned. By the third day, though, he still had a fever of 103 degrees, and he sounded very sleepy. At this point, I felt that he should see a doctor. Through friends, he contacted an emergency room attending physician who worked in one of the large local hospitals. The doctor had never seen my son, and obviously had never examined him, but he prescribed antibiotics for him over the telephone anyway. My son improved before he ever had a chance to take the antibiotics, but the moral of the story is that it is an error, a mistake, to prescribe over the telephone for a new patient who sounds sick and whom you have not even examined. My son probably had influenza, but he could have had anything, from pneumonia to meningitis.

And while we're on the subject of my family, here is what happened to my father, a retired ninety-year-old doctor. He had been on blood thinners for years when he developed some symptoms suggesting a problem with either his prostate or his bladder. A cystoscopy, a look into the bladder, was in order. Yet, because of the blood thinners, it was clear that no cutting could be done, since bleeding might result. The idea was just to see whether there was a problem that might need fixing at a later time.

When I came to see my father in his room several hours after the procedure, he was in severe pain. The location of the pain told me that urine was backed up in his bladder, and it was

214

obvious why: thick blood clots were blocking the catheter, the rubber pipe leading to the bladder. When I went out to the nurses' station to call his urologist, I looked at the chart. Right there, on the report of the cystoscopy, it said, "Resection of a small amount of prostatic tissue," or something very much like it. I do not know to this day whether the urologist forgot that my father was on blood thinners or whether he remembered and just took a chance in snipping off that little bit of prostate. Whatever his thinking, though, it was obvious that my father was bleeding heavily and that the reason for it was the ill-advised surgery done on a fully anticoagulated patient.

Luckily, I was able to find the urologist quickly. He came up and put a new catheter into the bladder, but my father had lost so much blood that he needed several transfusions. Ultimately he went home, but certainly he had been the victim of misprac-tice, which he did not need at his age, even though everything turned out all right in the end.

Where does mispractice end and malpractice begin? Is it the degree of the mistake that is important, or is it the outcome? True malpractice most usually involves bad judgment, and often goes hand in hand with carelessness and lack of knowl-edge. Mispractice suggests an only temporary lowering of the quality of what is done for the patient. Obviously, nothing is as important as a patient's life and health, but mispractice can be compared a little bit to the bad day that a chef has, or the three errors committed in one inning by the usually reliable short-stop. Yet the outcome also has a lot to do with whether we call it malpractice or mispractice. If my son had died, I would have considered the doctor's attitude negligent; as it was, I just con-sidered it stupid. If my father had died, I would have felt (rightly, I think) that the urologist was responsible for his death. If the lady in the recovery room had died, her family would have been entitled to think that malpractice had been committed. After all, in a major university hospital, it is reasonable to expect that, sooner or later, with fluids pouring into the patient's veins, *somebody* will wonder how much urine the patient is putting out and whether a bladder stretched by large amounts of urine is not at the bottom of the so far unexplained low blood pressure!

Doctors often make mistakes. Most of the time, though, that does not mean they are bad doctors. It just shows that they are human like the rest of us, prone to error and doubt. Unfortunately, mispractice cannot be erased altogether, so the next best thing is to try to prevent it as much as possible. We cannot promise that we will not make mistakes. That would be not only unrealistic but dishonest as well. What we can do, though, is make an all-out effort not to repeat these mistakes, and in this way lessen the likelihood of this all too human failing of ours.

It seems to me that patients are reluctant to accept the idea that errors are made in medicine, even in everyday practice. They have all heard about malpractice, but it often looks to them like something that only happens to somebody else, and what's more, that it is something that is larger than life, that it is not just a subtle, sometimes almost unnoticed, event. But for a doctor to make a mistake when he sees you in the office? Is it possible that he forgets to ask you whether you are allergic to penicillin when he prescribes for you a cephalosporin, a drug that can cause a reaction in penicillin-sensitive people? Yes, it is. And how about the doctor who is so busy that he forgets to ask whether you have ever had asthma when he gives you a prescription for a beta-blocker, a medication that can bring on an asthma attack in people who are prone to this condition? Most likely, these doctors usually take good care of you, and they will recognize that they have made a mistake if the patient has a bad reaction to their treatment. Not only will they recognize it, they are going to be so frightened by what they did, that devastating feeling of having *caused* an accident is going to be

216

so strong, that they are going to make adjustments in the way they practice for a long time to come.

If mispractice is all around us, and can happen at any time, shouldn't patients be doing their share to prevent it? Certainly doctors should carry full responsibility for their patients; after all, that is what they are trained for, and that is why we pay them. Yet can't we enlist patients and their families as their helpers, to cut down even further on the likelihood of something stupid and accidental creating a problem where none existed before?

My experience with doctors, nurses, hospitals—in other words, the whole health care process—is, of course, extensive, because I have spent so many years as part of it. But as I have grown older in medicine, I have learned to take less and less for granted. I am not worried about whether my patient is going to have a good coronary artery bypass operation. I know he will, because I know the quality of the work that is done in my hospital. But I can't guarantee that he won't be tripped up by the little things, like allergic reactions that can be prevented, urinary retention that is not considered, and oversedation that leads to pneumonia, to name just a few.

I have seen a lot of these mishaps happening to my patients, and of course, members of my own family have not escaped them, either. These experiences have made one thing clear to me: *Patients and their families must be more assertive!* That does not mean that they have to be belligerent or what the health care team likes to call "difficult," but they should serve notice that they are carefully watching what is being done to the patient.

Patients, if they are alert enough, should be taught to question all medications that are being given to them and to mention their allergies each time. If a patient "just doesn't look right," the relatives should look for a reason, and not just take it for granted that everybody else knows better than they do. What's more, if their instincts tell them that something serious is going on, they should insist on being allowed to stay in the hospital overnight, to see for themselves that the patient is receiving the best and most attentive care possible.

There is a fine line between hysteria and appropriate concern. Doctors can, often justifiably, become angry and defensive when they feel they are being questioned to death, and this, in turn, can work out to the disadvantage of the patient. Besides, doctors rightly feel that it is up to them to protect their patients from harm. Yet doctors are not there with the patient all the time, and he is not the only patient who requires their protection. This is why each sick person also needs an advocate, somebody who makes sure that he is getting a fair shake. Sometimes it is the patient himself who is the advocate, and sometimes it is a friend or a relative, but whoever it is, he is important in defending the patient against mispractice.

Suing after the fact is easy. There is something impersonal about having the lawyers slug it out, with the insurance company picking up the tab. Yet I would like to think that almost all patients would rather not have gone through the experience that brought about the suit. Money can never be an adequate reward for suffering; just ask the patients who have gone through pain, nausea, shortness of breath, tracheostomies, and the like. Unhappily, malpractice and mispractice are here to stay as long as imperfect people like us doctors lay hands on sickness-prone people like you patients. But the extent to which we mistreat you, and how often we do it, is still up to all of us. If we do our best to learn from our mistakes, can we count on you to always keep an eye on what we do to you?

11

Death

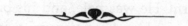

IN MEDICINE, death is never far from our thoughts. It is always there to remind us that there is an outer limit not only to what we can do but to the patient's capacity and will to live as well. Yet these are only abstract notions, and they do not touch on the emotional exchanges between our dying patients and us, our feelings after they have died, and the grave guilt that we experience when we realize that, for whatever reason, we did not do as much as we should have done to pull them back from the brink.

One of my first tours of duty during my internship was the emergency room. Before that, I had worked on one of the medical wards, where I was under the watchful and fatherly eye of a senior resident who taught me a lot, yet gave me very little responsibility. In contrast, the emergency room in those days was the province of the intern, who handled matters as he saw fit, called for consultation only when he really needed it, and referred the patient to the appropriate clinic for follow-up care when it was necessary.

After the first few days in my new little kingdom, I had already begun to feel comfortable treating colds, infected fingers, and urinary tract infections, the outermost reaches of an intern's unsupervised activities. I knew, of course, that I was going to be encountering much more complicated problems, but I kept hoping that they would come upon me at some time in the very distant future, when I would, I hoped, be much more knowledgeable.

One afternoon during my first week on the job, an elderly man with a long beard and wearing a skullcap at a slight tilt was helped in by two younger men who were supporting him, one under each arm. He was pale, and his black, shiny jacket was much too large for him. His voice was weak, and as he was saying a few words in Yiddish, while pointing to his stomach, the two younger men, who were evidently his sons, kept interrupting him, as well as each other. From what I could find out, the old man had had loss of appetite and abdominal pain for several weeks, and he had become weak and listless in the past several days. The fact that his jacket hung on him made sense to me. It meant that he had probably had a rapid, recent loss of weight, and the whole picture suggested to me a possible cancer of the stomach.

In the 1950s, a time when house calls were easy to obtain and finding a hospital bed was rarely a problem, the emergency room was usually a quiet place. Looking back on it, the pace was slower than it is nowadays, but because there were fewer patients, the cases were handled more quickly. Of course, we did not have AIDS in those days, and I worked in a private hospital, but even the more crowded facilities in city hospitals like Bellevue or Kings County did not approach the battlefield conditions that are considered to be normal today.

Nowadays, the emergency room has replaced the house call and, oftentimes, the function of the family doctor. Recently, though, it has also produced an offspring, the emergency ward. This is a holding area for patients who are too sick to be sent home but for whom there are no hospital beds available. With all these added functions, emergency rooms have become much too full, and patients often have to wait for hours just to be seen by a doctor. What's more, the overworked staff tries to give good care, yet it does not have the time to provide the emotional support that is so necessary for patients in this uncertain and frightening situation.

In the last few years of my practice, I did everything I could to keep my patients out of the emergency room. I tried either to admit them to the hospital directly or to take care of them at home for as long as possible, but there were times when I could not avoid this thoroughly unpleasant alternative. It is true that I felt much safer medically when a seriously ill patient was being watched and monitored while I investigated the possibility of a heart attack or a stroke, let us say. Yet the sight of patients lying around on stretchers in drafty hallways, the side rails perpetually up and suggesting individual little prisons, at a time when clean sheets and the armylike sense of order of a hospital means even more to the patient than the treatment he came in for, never failed to shock me. As a matter of fact, I was sometimes reminded of the scenes recorded during the Crimean War, where the wounded and sick suffered terribly in unspeakable surroundings. But I was outraged as well, because we have let budget considerations and allocation of hospital beds for bureaucratic rather than medical reasons interfere with the right of our citizens to be as comfortable and as tranquil as possible at the time when they need it most.

I had been warned by my fellow interns who had already served in the ER that patients would occasionally seek emergency care not necessarily because they were so sick but because it was easier and quicker to be seen there rather than in a doctor's office or in the clinic. The old man was obviously sick, but it seemed to me that the emergency room was not the place to investigate the cause. Yet, when I told his sons that I was referring him to the gastrointestinal clinic, which was meeting that afternoon, they were not satisfied with my decision. Both looked like younger (and healthier) versions of their father, and as I looked at them more closely, I realized that they were identical twins. To add to their resemblance, they wore their yarmulkes (skullcaps) at the same minimally rakish angle as their father did, although their gray beards were shorter than his, and the tight fit of their jackets could only suggest recent weight gain, rather than loss.

"If it says emergency room here, and our father looks and feels so terrible, isn't it an emergency? So why should we have to schlepp him somewhere else?" one of them objected, while the other, in an even louder voice, agreed with him. I tried my best to explain the purpose of the emergency room, that it was not a replacement for the clinic, and that he would get better care upstairs. They continued to argue, however, even threatening to call Rabbi Twersky, the powerful though unofficial Hasidic envoy to New York's medical community. But I became more resistant as they became more aggressive (I'm not going to give in to these Hasidim, I thought; I'd be the laughingstock of the hospital!). I finally cut the conversation short by having the patient put into a wheelchair, gave orders to send him upstairs, and then walked away as imperiously as I knew how.

Ten minutes later, I received an urgent call from the nurse in the clinic, who told me that my patient had fainted while being rolled upstairs and that they were sending him right back. When he arrived, he was obviously in shock, sweating profusely, with no obtainable blood pressure and a very rapid weak pulse. He also had about him the unmistakable smell of stool mixed with blood. After that, it all happened very quickly. He went into cardiac arrest and could not be resuscitated. I declared him dead no more than an hour after he had first arrived in the emergency room.

It did not require unusual medical wisdom to figure out what had happened. He was probably bleeding slowly (from an ulcer? from a cancer?), and that was the reason for his recent weakness. He must have had major blood loss (from his gastrointestinal tract, judging from the smell) while being taken upstairs, which caused him to go into shock and ultimately into cardiac arrest.

Of course, what I should have done was to evaluate the patient—that is, examine him and do some blood tests—before sending him to the clinic. If I had then kept him in the emergency room, put in an intravenous line, prepared to give him blood, and so on, and *not* wasted precious time in sending him to the clinic, I thought, maybe, just maybe, he might have been salvaged. I could not be certain that these maneuvers would have made the difference, but that is certainly what I thought then.

Despair is the right word for the overwhelming emotion that took hold of me. I had had an actual sinking physical sensation, that feeling of dread and terrible weakness that happens before a fainting spell, during the telephone conversation with the clinic nurse. After that, while we were trying to resuscitate the patient, I was too preoccupied to watch my own reactions. But when it was all over, and when I heard the loud crying of the sons who had dragged him in originally, I remember wishing that I could do the same thing, but even more, that I could scream my head off. At the same time, I had a crazy desire to throw myself on his body and beg his forgiveness. What's more, the sons had, of course, been right in not wanting to move him, and I had forced my judgment on them. I thought that I would rather die myself than have to face these two additional victims of mine ever again.

At that moment, I could not imagine continuing to be a doctor or even taking the slightest responsibility for another human being. All the doubts I might ever have had about going into medicine came to the surface, and in addition, I heaped on all my doubts about my person, my intelligence, and my powers of concentration. Yet I functioned well on another level. I filled out the chart, called the medical examiner, and did everything required of a doctor who has presided over a death. These clerical tasks helped to calm me down, and by this time my friends among the interns had begun to come around. I was not even surprised by their visits, because I was sure that by now all of New York had heard the news. They sat there with me, some dredging up stories of foul-ups in which they had been involved or that somebody had told them about, while others tried to convince me that my actions, however they appeared, had really been appropriate. But what my friends were really doing was giving emergency psychotherapy to the emergency room intern, certainly not a common occurrence, but one that helped to put me back on my feet.

Luckily, I was able to do the medical equivalent of climbing back into an airplane immediately after a crash. I managed to finish my shift and saw a few more patients, all of whom managed to leave the emergency room alive!

Of course, later in my training, by the time I had gotten more experience, I realized that I had not been responsible for the patient's death. I certainly could have handled the case more efficiently and more elegantly, but even if I had kept him in the emergency room, I doubted (and still do) that the few minutes of delay would have made the massive bleeding, the shock, and the cardiac arrest turn out differently.

Experience in medicine is often won at the expense of anxiety and uncertainty on the part of the doctor. The events I remember most are usually the ones that caused me the greatest anguish, as in this particular instance. Just remembering is not enough, though, and all the suffering by both patient and doctor should at least be of help to someone else down the line. Up to the episode with the old man, starting with my father's admonitions and continuing with medical school and the beginning of my internship, I had, of course, understood that we have an *obligation* to the patient to take as good care of him as is humanly possible. But what this episode, which put me

224

into such a state of emotional upheaval, taught me was that just providing good care is not enough. I had a glimmer of it then and became more and more convinced over the years of the notion that we have an even larger function to fulfill: we are responsible *for* our patients, and we must protect them as we do our own children, Our purpose is to give conscientious medical care, and we fulfill this purpose most of the time, but there are any number of incidents that happen to patients that can be avoided. The drug reaction, the anesthetic death, the oversedation, and so on sometimes occur because everybody goes by the book and nobody has that heightened awareness and that extra little bit of anxiety, as well as the momentary consideration of the worst-case scenario, that might well prevent a bad outcome.

I cannot put it in a better way, and I am not at all being patronizing when I say it, but I am certainly doing my duty by my patients if I send them across the street only when the light is green. But if I take the trouble to walk with them, and hold their hands in the bargain, then I am satisfying our highest calling, and that is the *shielding* of my patient from harm.

For the average person, death is an occasional intruder on his consciousness. It may be a relative or a friend who has died, and often it is someone close enough so that the sorrow is deep and long lasting. But still, it does not happen often, and periods of mourning usually do not overlap.

For us, doctors who take care of patients until the very end, death is familiar, not that the familiarity makes us any less terrified of it. There is an almost predictable incidence of it in patients with severe heart disease, cancer, and so on, and in addition, there are the "sudden" deaths, those that were not "expected." These always make the conscientious doctor ask himself questions, often in the middle of the night, about whether he missed anything that might have been a clue to the development of the ultimate tragedy. But expected or unexpected, predictable or not, a patient's death commonly touches doctors very emotionally. In an active practice, like mine, for example, there was almost always someone dying or someone who had just died. There was never really a respite from it, so there was always some corner of me that was in mourning. I still miss, some after years and years, many of the patients who died while under my care, and it seems to me, and this may just be imagination, that I have lost many of those I liked best. It is possible that they seem dearer to me than they did in life only when I look back. Whatever the truth is, though, I am often reminded of one or another dead patient of mine, and I think of almost all of them fondly.

Doctors' responses to patients' deaths are open to misinterpretation because, as is so often the case with us, we keep our feelings to ourselves. This is understandable, however, because we have a responsibility to the survivors to be calm and reassuring, to explain what happened, and not to join in demonstrations of grief. But where we often fail is in not at *some* time giving to ourselves and to the families an indication of how we felt about the patient and, possibly, how much we will miss him.

Instead, we go back to our macho role, where nothing touches us or gets beneath our "professional" exterior. Of course, we must protect ourselves to some degree, and we cannot obsess about each patient's death; otherwise the care of our surviving patients would suffer. Yet at the same time, we cannot act as if nothing out of the ordinary happened, because there is no question that it did. Just being somebody's doctor, even if the person is not sick, brings up recollections beyond diagnoses, laboratory tests, and so on. But if the patient is sick enough to die, should that not produce an untold number of remembrances, many of which are poignant enough to break first into, and then out of, our self-imposed shell?

My father tells me what his grandmother used to tell him: "Every doctor has his own little cemetery." I am not sure what she meant by that when she said it at the beginning of this century. Maybe doctors of that time, with what looks to us now like primitive knowledge, and lacking any truly effective drugs, were responsible for enough deaths to stock a small or even medium-size cemetery. But I choose to use my great-grandmother's saying for my own purposes. I have frequently, in my mind, walked up and down the lanes of *my* cemetery, where my patients are buried. I have stopped in front of this or that name and remembered some distinctive little mannerism that endeared the patient to me. Or I was reminded of some very early morning encounter in the intensive care unit, when the patient's dying and my desperate maneuvers to keep him alive merged totally into one entity. At that moment, it seemed to me that nothing else in the world was of any importance to us, just our interaction. We were closer than husband and wife, or parents and children. He was hanging out the window, and only my hand grip kept him from falling. But I could not lift him back, and our grips became weaker and weaker. We finally had to let go, but I will never forget either his falling or my sense of terrible helplessness at not being able to hold on.

Enid McNally was my patient for about twenty years. She had rheumatic heart disease, and when I first saw her, when she was about fifty, she already had an irregular heart rhythm and fluid in her lungs. Because her condition did not respond adequately to medication, she had a mitral valvuloplasty, a repair of one of her heart valves that had been damaged by her childhood rheumatic fever. She was much better after the operation and was able to continue in her work as an executive for the Girl Scouts. Soon after her surgery, she was asked to retire because of a reorganization of her office, and I asked (actually pleaded) with her to take charge of my practice. She worked with me for about fifteen years, and we got along beautifully. She was an angular, tall woman of Scotch-Irish origins who was a great baseball fan, played the piano beautifully, and was probably the only executive secretary in the neighborhood who had graduated from the Sorbonne. What's more, I knew she had made a hit with my patients when, early on, they would call the office and, when I accidentally picked up the phone, would say, "Dr. Berczeller, I don't want to speak to you. Could you please get Enid for me?" Yet she could be tough when she wanted to be. Even I became frightened sometimes when her manner would suddenly change. Her speech became clipped, all the kidding was gone, and I knew that a patient was being told that he had gone too far in some demand or some complaint having to do with office business.

Enid, of course, continued to be my patient after she started working for me; as a matter of fact, she laughingly used to refer to this as one of her "perks." We would go through the formality of having regular appointments. At those times, she would call the answering service to answer our phones, take her chart out of the file drawer and hand it to me, and then go into the examining room to put on a gown. Even though we were by this time on a first-name basis, she invariably called me Dr. Berczeller while she was being examined, and in contrast to our usual joking with each other, we both behaved in a very sober manner during these monthly visits. Over the years, her condition again worsened. At first, her breathlessness and palpitations responded to a change or an increase in her medications, but by the mid-1980s it became clear to both of us that she could no longer continue working. On her last day, when we said good-bye, we were both crying. I was inconsolable; after all, I was losing my right hand! But she managed to see the bright side. "That's the only good thing about being sick," she said. "Even though I'm getting rid of this obnoxious job, I can still see you whenever I want!" Over the next few years, her heart failure worsened. I often considered another open-heart operation for her, this time with replacement of the mitral valve, but I was afraid to risk it because of her poor circulation and diminished lung function, both aggravated by her heavy smoking, which she refused to stop. Finally, the medications no longer did anything for her. I knew that she would die if she did not have an immediate operation. Yet her other medical problems were so severe that it was questionable whether she would survive the postoperative period, let alone ultimately be able to leave the hospital.

Doctors in a sense welcome the need to explain, to patient and family, their reason for recommending a particular procedure. In this way, some of the responsibility is taken off their shoulders, and if something goes wrong, the decision was at least made with everyone's consent. Yet with Enid, I did not even have this comfort. When I explained to her how serious her situation really was, and what my qualms were about having her operated on, she said, "Peter, even if John [her husband] were still alive, I would still do exactly what *you* recommend. I've depended on you ever since I met you, and I know that you'll keep me going, whatever you decide!" I guess there was no real choice. It was certain death against certain postoperative complications, so I bit the bullet. She survived the operation but spent the next five months in the intensive care unit. She had infections, she had heart failure, she had disturbances in her heart rhythm, her lung function was terrible, and she needed a tracheostomy (a hole in her windpipe) to breathe in adequate amounts of oxygen. What's more, she was disoriented much of the time, a not unusual event in the ICU, where there is no day and no night, only around-the-clock activity, just like in Las Vegas. Afterward, once she was home, she told me that she had no recollection at all of those months in the ICU, except that she remembered my frequently bending over her, pounding her on the back, and yelling, "Enid, cough, God damn it!" (Generally accurate, but maybe a little exaggerated, on thinking back.) Yet she said that she had not been shocked by my manner, since it was not that different from the temperamental way I behaved in the office. (Now her memory is becoming too good, I thought.)

I saw her at home on the day before I left for my vacation in July 1991. Her breathing had been steadily improving and maybe it was because, as she claimed, she had stopped smoking. After her original discharge from the hospital, she had fallen and broken a vertebra, so she had some difficulty in walking, but in general, although all my fears about postoperative complications had come true, the operation had clearly helped her. She was, as usual, sitting in her favorite easy chair, watching her cherished New York Mets. Although I did not see any cigarettes, there was a hint of stale smoke in the air, but I decided not to make an issue of it. I did not want her to feel disapproved of by me, especially just before I was leaving. A glass containing a pale yellow liquid stood within reaching distance. She had told me long ago that the frequent drinking of this substance was for her an irreplaceable link with her Scotch heritage. Since it obviously did her some good, I was glad to see that her reverence for tradition had not changed over the years.

I examined her, gave her instructions about her medications, and made sure she knew who was going to take care of her in my absence. This was the first time since her surgery that I was going to be away for any length of time, and I knew very well that she was concerned about it. I told her again how well she had done and that I expected her to improve even more as time went on. She replied that she believed me, that she never doubted anything I told her, but that she felt truly safe only if I was nearby—"or at least on this side of the ocean." I reassured her that the office would always be able to reach me, wherever I was in Europe, if she needed me. Looking back on it, though, I feel that she considered me some sort of good-luck charm that had kept her going for all those years. Now I understand much better why my nearness gave her such relief.

Before I kissed her good-bye, I gave her her staying-home present, tapes of the string quartets of her favorite composer, Schubert. She said, "Aren't you nice," pulled my head down to give me an extra thank-you kiss, and that was that.

Enid's successor, Marian, has never been known to keep unusual news to herself, and has called me in some remote places to give me information that could safely have waited for me until I got home. Since I received no calls from Marian, and since Enid had been in relatively good shape when I left, I was not unduly worried about her. Yet she was very much on my mind on the flight back from Europe, to the point where I felt a growing impatience to speak to her as soon as possible.

The morning after my arrival, when I woke up, it was much too early to call Enid, so I started to read the *New York Times*, which had already been delivered. I usually look at the obituaries after I read the sports section, and there was Enid's death announcement. She had evidently died a few days before, and the burial had already taken place, in the family plot in Maine.

It was around six o'clock in the morning, and it would be several hours before I could call anyone—that is, the doctor who covered for me, or Marian—to find out what had happened. In the meantime, the tranquillity that a month away from work usually brings to me had abruptly disappeared. This had happened to me before, this business of unexpected deaths during my vacation, I thought, as the realization that I would never see Enid again began to sink in. Edie, my first patient ever in private practice, had died several years before, also in August, while I was away. And Robert Rieger, a charming old psychoanalyst, had not kept his promise a few years before that when he said to me in typical Viennese bittersweet style, "Don't worry, I'll never give anyone else but you the pleasure of watching me die," and proceeded to die suddenly just five days before my return from another one of those damned vacations!

Of course, I would have been no less upset with the deaths of these people even if I had been with them until the very end. But I would at least have felt some relief, because of my realization that I had done my personal best to keep them alive. It was not that I did not trust the people who substituted for me. It was, rather, that a belief that is certainly not unique and that I share with many of my colleagues would have been satisfied, and that is that I (and in their case, they) can do just a little better than the next physician. What's more, in this kind of situation, even though there is an obvious finality attached to the patient's death, there is no finality to the doctor's sense of responsibility for him. Instead, there is only a gradual petering out of this feeling, which, at least for me, makes for a sense of emptiness that takes a long, long time to go away.

In Enid's case, I used the couple of hours before official life began in New York for toting up all the things I could feel guilty about. Why did I not call her from Europe? Maybe she would have told *me* something that would have indicated some change in her condition. This woman had depended on me so much. Was it right for me to leave her? Did I give the covering doctor all the information he needed? After all, her case was complicated, and maybe I forgot to tell him something important.

Actually, Enid's death was due to an accident. She had evidently been doing well until she fell once more. Because of the fall, she had pain in the chest on breathing, which led to a collapse of part of her lung, and she ultimately died because of respiratory failure. In other words, this time there was no way to improve the function of her lungs the way we did after the operation. I felt a little less guilty after I heard about the events leading up to her death, but then I began more and more to feel that familiar sense of loss, the mourning of which I have already spoken. Strangely enough, I was able to separate the feelings I had for her as a patient from the ones I had about her as a co-worker. I realized that the mourning had to do mainly with the patient part of Enid, with whom I had such intimate contact and who thought of me as her good-luck charm.

After so many years of being a doctor and witnessing the deaths of so many of my patients, I think it was Enid's death that gave me an additional insight, although it only came to me maybe a year later. I realized then that we not only miss the patient, in other words, his presence, after he is gone. What we miss also, and probably even more, is the individual relationship we had with the patient, that particular interaction that is as unique as a fingerprint and that will never come our way again.

Just as members of the family, each in their individual way, must begin to say good-bye to the patient when his death seems both inevitable and imminent, so the doctor also has to prepare himself emotionally for what is about to happen. On some level, we doctors very likely believe in the totally unrealistic notion that we *can* prevent death and that for some reason or other we were not skillful enough or caring enough to be successful in the particular case of *this* patient who is about to die. Of course, it is our ever-present guilt that is speaking, and we translate this guilt into our usually confused agenda of when and how to let the patient finally die. Patients and their families are understandably also uncertain about when to "pull the plug," so these conflicts on both sides of the bed make decision making in this emotionally overcrowded territory a very unstable proposition.

Ernestine Heller, an elderly Austrian-born longtime patient of mine, was clearly very desperately ill. She had an aggressive form of leukemia, unfortunately very different from the more benign type much more commonly seen in her age group. Months before, when she had still been moderately comfortable, though aware of her diagnosis, we had agreed that I would not engage in any life-saving heroics "when the time comes." (This was at a time before formal living wills became popular, but—and this may be a revelation to many in this legalistic age—doctors and patients have been known for centuries to have great mutual trust and to consider their verbal agreements binding.) She lay in her hospital bed, very short of breath and repeatedly coughing up blood. What's more, there were little reddish blue spots of hemorrhage under her skin everywhere on her body.

Her outlook was obviously terrible. She had not responded to any of the drugs used to combat this type of leukemia, and now it was no longer a question of if, but just when, she would die. On this particular day, I felt that the last, most helpful, thing that I could do for her in view of her terrible suffering was to live up to our agreement and to do nothing extraordinary from then on to keep her alive. I told her of my conclusion as gently as I could, in that calm and reassuring manner we doctors pull out of our hats at times like these. Yet, just underneath the manner, I felt, as I always did in this situation, the unavoidable horror that any human being *must* experience when announcing to the condemned that his death sentence is to be carried out without further delay.

Despite her distress, she was, as usual, extraordinarily alert. She asked me to prop her up on several pillows—her own, by the way, and embroidered with her initials, "E.H." "Herr Doktor," she said (we always spoke in German, which was our common mother tongue), "can't we just try it for one more day?" Of course we could, I replied, without going into useless reminders about long-ago agreements. I immediately made arrangements to continue with the ritual of blood transfusions, antibiotics, blood gases, and the like. We shook hands, and I promised to see her again before going home, early in the evening.

Listening for the location of the "airway" (a brief term for all the maneuvers used in an attempted resuscitation), or "code," when it is urgently broadcast at least three times in a row over the hospital loudspeaker (What do the telephone operators feel when they have to announce these catastrophic events? I have sometimes thought) is so imbedded in someone like myself who has dealt with patients every day for so long that I automatically listen for it even when I make a social call on a patient in a hospital not my own.

Whenever I had a patient who was barely hanging on to his life, I listened more carefully than ever for exactly where the airway was taking place. Sometimes the suspense was relieved quickly, because if the airway was called, let us say, for 16 West, and I had no patient on that floor, that meant that both my critically ill patient and I had at least had a momentary reprieve. If I did have a patient on the unit that was called out, though, and especially if he was very sick, I would try my best to look as unconcerned as possible, but would still go up to that particular floor while hoping that the airway cart was not in front of my patient's room. I admit freely that we doctors have a battlefield mentality at those times. We know very well that war kills, but we want our specific patient to be spared by the bullet flying in his general direction.

Toward the end of my rounds, and a few minutes before I was going to go to see Mrs. Heller again, an airway was called.

It was for 17 West, her floor, and this time I did not even go to the trouble of appearing nonchalant. I ran up the stairs, and when I reached her unit, the crash cart was standing in front of her door, and the number of people running in and out of her room confirmed my worst fears. She would have to go through an attempted resuscitation before being allowed to die! I realized, of course, that if we had agreed to give up earlier in the afternoon and if I had not felt pushed to restart her treatment, she would probably have died quietly, without fuss. But the blood transfusions and antibiotics and drawing of blood gases had sent the wrong signal to the nurses and residents. They probably thought that if she was being treated so intensively she could be salvaged as well.

It has to be understood that an airway unfolds like a classical tragedy. Once it is started, it has to continue until either the patient shows evidence (rising blood pressure, effective rhythm of the heart, and so on) of coming back to life or until it is obvious that he is truly dead and that no amount of mechanical assistance is likely to make the difference. There is no way an airway can be stopped in the middle, even if it is obvious, as it was in this case, that it was a useless exercise that would only prolong the patient's suffering. No physician would take the chance of stopping an attempt to restore a patient's life. The hospital authorities would strongly disapprove, and almost certainly the doctor would end up being sued by somebody.

I have often been horrified by the violent nature of the death of patients in the hospital. The last view that these people often have of the world is of a pack of euphoric youngsters slapping on electrodes and yelling for medications, in short, confronting a stranger's emergency. When I witness these scenes (I say "witness" because as a doctor trained in the 1950s I find it best to stay on the sidelines of these high-tech exercises), usually sitting on the radiator, my personal observation balloon, I sometimes think about that institution of bygone centuries, the deathbed, and how people were allowed to die in that bed with their families around them. The patient lay on his back, the bed was crisply made, his arms were neatly stretched over the coverlet, and when the death rattle came, there was no attempt to squeeze another few minutes or days out of a waning life.

Yet nowadays, possibly because we have been lured into a false sense of power by our ability to tame a small part of our environment just a little bit, we are especially frustrated and impatient with the unchanging, and resistant, nature of death. So we have changed dying from a ceremony into a torture. It is true that, especially in recent times, living wills and health care proxies have helped a great deal in preventing some of us from resuscitating *everybody*, regardless of their hopeless outlook. In addition, there is a strong case to be made against what amounts to cruelty to the dying, who are subjected to "codes" that prolong life for only minutes or hours, or produce a comatose, intubated patient whose basic disease is bound to kill him very soon anyway.

Yet what do we know, those of us who are not old or who do not have a life-threatening illness? Can we be the true spokesmen for our future incarnations at the point of death? Does anyone really know what the dying experience? Don't they all feel terror at what is to befall them? Aren't there at least some who echo Mrs. Heller's plea to stay with the only game in town, life, for another day?

12

Finding the Right Doctor

IN THE EYES OF our patients, what do we doctors lack most? Many say that we lack empathy, but is this really what they want from us? Giving a definition of the qualities that patients expect us to possess is not just an exercise in language. It is, rather, an opportunity to explore how far their expectations are realistic, and how capable we are of fulfilling them.

Is it better for the patient if I project myself *into* what he is experiencing? Don't I then take on his feelings, and in the meantime lose my objectivity? Do I have to talk myself into sharing the patient's shortness of breath or pain in order to effectively treat these distressing symptoms? Does empathy really fit in with what is already our deepest obligation, the relief of our patients' suffering?

I think that sympathy is a much more appropriate emotion for us to feel toward our patients. It means that we have solidarity with them, that we have pity for them, and that we do not leave their side as we feel *along* with them. At the same time, though, it allows us to keep that distance which is so necessary if we are to look at the patient and his problem soberly. In other words, sympathy allows us to do what we are supposed to do, as well as to use our best judgment, while taking a step back in order to look at the total picture more clearly.

Yet I don't think most people bother their heads too much

about whether it is empathy or sympathy they want from their doctors. Instead, they want to know that he *cares*, that they are much more than just a chart, or an interesting case, or a source of income for him. Certainly they want technical competence, but I am convinced that emotional warmth from the person who is supposed to be their guide around the frightening labyrinth that houses sickness and medicine is at least equally important.

When I was in training, I could not understand sometimes why certain doctors who were not considered too bright by us young hot shots had such busy practices. I remember one in particular, let's call him Sam Tauber. We used to refer to his patients as "Sam's marines" because they would do only what Sam, or someone who dropped his name, would tell them to do. Each new group of residents would find this out rather quickly, so if we wanted a patient of his to submit to anything from a laxative to an x-ray, "Dr. Sam wants it right away" was the open sesame. Meanwhile, Sam was anything but a hero to his fellow attending physicians or to us trainees. He was so unsure of himself that he could never make up his mind, and he constantly asked for advice not only from his peers but also from us medical children. Yet, he caused no harm that I can remember, probably especially because, in his insecurity, he called for multiple consultations on each patient and finally did what the majority suggested. Yet his patients only saw the side of him that cared enough to call for the second (and third, and fourth, and so on) opinions. He sat with them while the consultant was examining them, and always came back afterward with at least a tiny piece of good news wrapped in a cheerful smile. Of course, we rough-and-ready fledgling paratroopers, who believed only in the absolute truths that medicine had to teach us and in the importance of quick decision making (never mind whether the decisions turned out to be right or wrong), referred to Sam as an "old lady." Yet it was good to have him around, not only because he was great comic relief but also because we always felt much smarter than we really were after he stopped us in the hall and asked *us*, the lowest of the low, for an opinion on some patient of his who was not doing well.

There are pitifully few advantages to getting older, but certainly one of them is that you learn to know better. Nowadays, of course, I realize that you do not have to be a genius to be a doctor. I do not deny that it is exhilarating (because it has, fortunately, happened to me) to make correct diagnoses of unusual conditions though the clues are minimal, or to come up with the right treatment despite advice to the contrary from a corps of consultants. Some of us live for that high, which comes up only occasionally in a medical lifetime. I was even worse in sports than Dr. Sam was in medicine, so I don't know how it feels to hit a home run with the bases loaded, or to score the winning basket with no time left. But I imagine that it must be something like that flash of insight that happens much too infrequently for those of us who are hooked on it and that is even more precious and memorable because it is so rare. Yet to provide human warmth—and not only to care greatly but to *show* the patient that you care—is a talent in itself. Sam Tauber gave great comfort to his patients, and in the long run did much good, despite his insecurity and his lack of judgment.

I spoke of distance before, and the need to step back. But one of the crucial misunderstandings between patients and doctors has to do with *how far* the doctor has to step back in order to do his job while still not surrendering his humanity. No matter how much compassion we have for the patient's suffering, there is still a wide gulf between what the patient experiences and what we feel when we witness it. Many different emotions intrude upon my consciousness when I sit with a patient who is moaning with pain like a sick animal, or one who is terribly agitated about an upcoming operation.

Certainly, I am genuinely touched by what my fellow human being is going through. But at the same time, I am busily thinking about how best to stop the pain, or what to say to relieve, even a little bit, the fear of "going under" that the patient who is first on the next day's operating schedule is experiencing. I also feel frustrated because I know that even if I stop it now, the patient's pain will come back soon, and that, whatever I say, the upcoming night will still be agonizing for tomorrow's first surgical candidate.

And then there is my divided attention when I am faced with an emergency. Let's say the patient has pulmonary edema (water on the lungs). His lips are blue, he obviously has a great deal of difficulty in breathing, and he is very frightened and agitated because of the terrifying sense of asphyxiation he must be feeling. As I am thinking of what to give him, and how much, I hold his hand and tell him that he will feel much better as soon as the medication we are about to give him starts working. But I am also distracted by practical matters. He obviously belongs in the ICU; how soon can I get a bed there? When is that damn x-ray technician going to come to do the portable chest x-ray? Is the patient's blood pressure going to hold up when, as I hope, he starts pouring out urine in response to the medication? Which reminds me: we have to put a catheter into his bladder so that we can measure his output accurately. In the meantime, I at least figuratively hold on to his hand and report whatever good news I can find. The 100 percent oxygen he is breathing from a mask has made him a little pinker, and I tell him so. In the meantime, he has gotten some morphine, he is quieter, and I ask the nurse to call for the results of the latest arterial blood gas to see whether it reflects the small improvement I think I detect clinically.

Out of the corner of my eye, I have once or twice seen the frightened faces of his wife and daughter at the door (this all

241

happened during visiting hours), and I take a couple of minutes to go out and talk to them, leaving the resident and intern to watch the patient.

In these situations, we doctors are in a terrible dilemma. Certainly we should never show fear or panic to the patient or his family, because this can only increase the anxiety they are already feeling. Yet if we appear casual in our attempt to shield them, at least temporarily, from frightening truths, we are said to be "unfeeling" or "cold technicians." Of course, we can be more honest with relatives than with the patient who is critically ill with an oxygen mask tightly clamped to his face, but even the information given to the family under these circumstances has to be screened very carefully. Relatives sometimes have a way of immediately transmitting to the patient unpleasant information given to them in confidence. Yet even if nothing is said, the average patient can certainly draw his own conclusions if he sees a whole bunch of crying relatives gathered around his bed, even as they deny to him, as if in one voice, that there is anything wrong.

I spent the several minutes that I could spare in explaining to his wife and daughter what had happened. I played up the fact that he seemed to be getting better, and although I mentioned that he could possibly worsen again, I did not go into my experiences with pulmonary edema. This condition is notoriously treacherous and had caused quite a few deaths in my patients, especially during the earlier years of my practice, before the powerful diuretics became available.

I would say that my attitude in this case was halfway between very concerned and casual. As it turned out, the patient improved, and my middle approach turned out to have been appropriate. But what if the patient had had a cardiac arrest soon after my conversation with his family? Might they not have been angry at me afterward for appearing *too* casual as I ambled out to talk to them or as I kidded around a little bit

242

with the patient and with the staff? Or what if his clinical situation and the blood gases had not improved or even gotten worse, which would have made me even more concerned than I already was? I might then have paid less attention to both actual and figurative hand-holding because pestering the ICU to speed up the transfer, arranging for the placement of a Swan-Ganz catheter, and so on, would have taken up all my attention in my attempt to keep him alive. Under these circumstances, I might well have warned the family that he could possibly die. But if he had finally improved, might he not have complained then that I was a humorless technician when he needed reassurance most and, what's more, that I had needlessly "scared the hell" out of his wife and daughter?

In medicine, and especially at critical times, what the patient or his family sees is frequently *not* what there is. When what we know about the patient and his illness is mixed in with our medical knowledge and experience, the end product, we hope, is good judgment, something we all strive for. It is easy to dismiss what a doctor advises by saying, "It just doesn't make sense!" or to be miffed by a change in his behavior in the middle of a serious situation. Yet most of the time there is a logic to what we do. What can be so misleading is that it is *not* the logic of everyday life, and it can therefore easily appear bizarre to our patients.

Obligation between doctors and patients seems to us to be a one-way street. In other words, as professionals we are bound by our sense of duty and code of ethics to take care of our patients. On the other hand, though, there are no rules that govern how patients behave toward us, so it is perfectly permissible for them to come and go and act as they please, which is very much out of keeping with the heavy responsibility that we carry for them.

But sympathy should be a two-way street between our patients and us. While we are learning to be more sensitive to the complaints our patients have against us, it would genuinely help the relationship if we sensed that they had some understanding of what we go through. If they felt along with us (as many of us try to do with them), they might then give us a little more leeway and try to make sense of what we are doing, rather than judging us prematurely. I know it is difficult for them to imagine (with their fantasies of how we hold all the cards) how much the tone of the doctor-patient relationship depends on them as well as on us. But then again, we doctors are no different from other people. Like them, we are grateful for an expression of encouragement, a pat on the back, and a sign of appreciation for our efforts. At the same time, though, we resent, as does any self-respecting horse, the needless use of the whip when we are already running as fast as we can.

Some doctors take a larger step back than others, but most of the time, it seems to me, they can still convince their patients of their interest and caring. Yet there is an enormous distance between what we measure in steps and that dreary and discouraging territory that is the province of the remote doctor. These people have permanently shut off, for whatever emotional reasons of their own, any sense of pity or understanding for the patient's problem. Many of these doctors, probably through a process of self-screening, know enough about themselves to go into fields that require no patient contact at all, like research, or into specialties such as pathology or radiology, for example, where they can communicate results to another physician who then interacts with the patient. (It goes without saying, of course, that there are many doctors in the fields I just mentioned who have excellent patient skills and who chose these areas for reasons having nothing to do with emotion.)

Unfortunately, sometimes the screening process fails, and the uncaring individual with poor insight stumbles into an area where compassion for the patient is a must. This can be a catastrophe, and the patient is, as would be expected, the victim.

Jeff is easily one of the most gifted people ever to come out of our surgical training program. I admit it; we internists used to look at surgeons as two hands with a brain attached as an afterthought, a judgment that cannot really be sustained these days, what with sophisticated organ transplant procedures and increasingly complicated cardiac surgery. Twenty-five years ago, though, when Jeff was a rotator on our medical internship at Bellevue, my senior attending and I paid him, in our elitism and smugness, the highest compliment we could think of: "Jeff is good enough to go into internal medicine!" At that time, I was not particularly struck by his personality, either way, and I expected that somewhere down the line, after he was finished with his training, I would start referring patients to him. Surgical residents are like ghosts. They vanish into the operating room for days, or disappear to do research for years at a time, so it did not strike me as unusual not to have contact with Jeff again until about fifteen years ago. When he came to my attention, though, I was not happy with what I saw or heard. It was not only that he never returned my greeting or even acknowledged my existence when we met, which would have been par for the course for surgeons recently out of their training who had not yet learned how to deal with adult doctors in other specialties but was distinctly unusual for anyone whose teacher I had been. What really bothered me, though, was what I heard from several sources, and that was that some of the families of patients who had been operated on by Jeff complained bitterly to the referring physicians about him. This was extraordinary in itself, because patients and their families, as if in repayment for a successful operation by a top surgeon, are willing to take a lot of nonsense, including long delays in the scheduling of the surgery, delegation of most communication to the resident, and so on. But for not one but several families to go on the warpath required more than the usual annoyances, and I was curious to know what they were. By this time word had reached me that Jeff, although relatively junior in rank and in experience, was already recognized as an innovative, fearless, and technically superb operator. This in itself would have stimulated me to send some of my patients to him, but what I heard about his human relations made me very cautious. Over the next several weeks, I found out what I wanted to know. It seemed that Jeff did not want to communicate with families at all, that he brushed them off when he encountered them in the hall and he did not return their phone calls. The patients themselves also complained of getting very little information out of him, and what's more, the referring physicians, with the exception of a chosen few, were also given the cold shoulder. Regretfully, I knew then that, despite his great talent, I could never work with him. I am notoriously quick on the trigger myself and also very sensitive to how my patients are treated by my colleagues. In addition, the niceties of behavior between doctors are important to me, so I knew that Jeff and I would be at each other's throats immediately if I were ever to send a patient to him. But what convinced me more than ever that he is truly remote is an episode I witnessed a few years ago.

Jeff had operated on Henry Green, an elderly member of our staff, someone who had been around for many years and who came from a generation of surgeons in which bedside manner was still held in great esteem. The operation had gone well, but Henry had respiratory complications after surgery, needed a tracheostomy, and ultimately ran into feeding problems. I used to see him in the ICU and, afterward, in the hall of one of the regular patient floors when I was making rounds, and it was very obvious that he was failing. He was very thin (by this time he had a gastrostomy, a hole in his stomach for feeding purposes), and he could speak only if he placed a finger over the tracheostomy tube. But he still managed to look urbane, sitting there in his Sulka dressing gown with a silk polka dot scarf around his neck that he parted slightly when he wanted to speak.

When we meet up with fellow doctors who are patients in the hospital, it is sometimes very difficult to know how to behave toward them. Do you just greet them pleasantly and then go on, not wishing to intrude on their privacy? Or do you show interest by asking about their illness, and in the process possibly disturb the delicate balance between what they have been told, what they know, and what they want to know? In his case, though, there was really no mystery or suspense, since his appearance gave away his entire story. I would sometimes sit with him for a few minutes, and we would chat about some of the interesting cases we had seen together over the years, never forgetting to mention the drama surrounding the very painful (and initially puzzling) appearance of a herpes on my mother's right index finger. I say "chat" but it was really I who chattered while he occasionally made a comment in that sepulchral, disembodied voice so typical of patients with tracheostomies. One day, as I was just getting ready to leave, the surgeons advanced upon us. It is not coincidental that they travel in packs (called "teams"), what with their large numbers and the wave of sound that regularly announces their arrival. Very much like a part of some military maneuver, each cohort was distinguished by a color, and this was, if I remember correctly, the blue team. Even without a scorecard, I was able to identify the players. First of all there was Jeff, in a scrub gown and cap, which gave the impression (possibly studied?) of his having just this moment stepped away from the operating table. Then there was the fellow, the top sergeant, who had finished his surgical residency and was Jeff's subspecialty trainee. I had virtually never seen this position filled by anyone but a tall, taciturn, brusque individual with a southern accent, and this one was no different. The rest of the group was made up of eight people carrying clipboards. I knew from experience that some of them were students (probably the four who hung slightly behind and who were not spoken to at all) and the rest were the residents and interns, the human computer screens who lent their voices to the laboratory, x-ray, and consultation results that were constantly being accumulated by and then spit forth from those insatiable clipboards.

Henry's wife, his two sons, and I stood around Henry's wheelchair, and although there was no sign of recognition from anyone in the advancing little army, it seemed that they had come to visit him, since they stopped in front of us. The fellow asked, "Howya doin', Doc?" but before the old surgeon could activate his voice by sticking his finger on the tracheostomy opening, the fellow was already interrogating one of the clipboard bearers on the day's "numbers." They did not really examine Henry, but the report must have been satisfactory, since its very telling had transmitted marching orders to the little troop. Jeff had not said a word to patient, family, or visitor, and now turned around to walk out, offering us a half wave of his hand as he did so. Henry's older son had just been telling me that he had called Jeff at least twice daily for a week to get an update on his father's condition, but that he had never received a reply. He now ran after Jeff and caught up to him just as the team was walking out the door of the room. He then spoke so quietly that I could not hear what he said. There was no mistaking Jeff's shouted reply, though, since we all, including Henry, heard it very clearly. "Look, there's no use calling all the time! He's not going to get better than this. What you see is what there is!"

From what I could see, his judgment was correct. Henry died a few days later, as if to indicate his agreement, good old clinician that he was, with his younger colleague's assessment of the situation. But Jeff's behavior, which I had now seen at first hand, convinced me that no amount of technical skill or even genius can justify what finally has to be recognized as cruel behavior toward patients and their families.

Patients often asked me, when I was referring them to a particular specialist, whether I would send someone from my family to him. I invariably replied that it would be unthinkable for me to use different consultants for them and for my relatives. If I were to choose a doctor for my patients, my children, my wife, my parents, or for myself, I would always try to find someone who is a combination of the *good* qualities of Sam Tauber and Jeff—in other words, kindness combined with competence. On paper, the ideal doctor would strike a perfect balance between the willingness and ability to provide emotional support to his patients and the capacity to use his large fund of knowledge for their benefit. I have never met any doctors who have this ideal mix in real life, so I have had to be satisfied with people who at least try to combine a sense of humanity and humaneness with technical skill. I think that patients are helped if they have doctors who realize that there is always room for improvement in their own performance. A doctor's occasional insecurity and uncertainty, far from being a disadvantage, can actually be very helpful to the patient. There is no such thing as certainty in medicine. Any doctor who is "absolutely sure" of a diagnosis or who feels that "there is no question" that a treatment will work doesn't know what he is talking about and should be avoided. I have always said that the doctor I respect most is one who is not a genius but instead worries a lot, and I guess I personally fulfill that job description. We doctors worry for our patients because we know how bad it can be out there and that we constantly risk being blindsided by the incalculable nature of life or of the environment. Patients worry for themselves as well, and for identical reasons. This merging of our worries cannot help but produce a strong link between us, and should help, even a little, to dispel the patients' perennial notion that "doctors just don't care."

Surprisingly, one of the most important issues in the relationship between doctors and patients is regularly overlooked, and it is this: DOCTORS HAVE TEMPERAMENTS! Their responses to stress, to illness, and to situations that arouse their pity; their feelings about life and death; even the field of medicine that they go into; all these are under the control of that characteristic and unique way of looking at the world that is the individual temperament. Certainly we have to try to take the patient's temperament into account if we hope to gain his cooperation and at the same time hit the right note when we try to explain his illness to him. But what makes doctors tick has always remained a mystery to patients, and although patients have always recognized that, let us say, some of us are "quiet" and others "have a lot of personality," I do not believe that many have understood how far-reaching doctors' personality traits really are and how much of an effect they have on the care that the patient receives.

And yet, should patients not recognize us much more easily than they do? After all, we come from the same emotional backgrounds as theirs. We are not brought up in some priestly sect where all the "good" and "right" things are programmed into us from earliest childhood. As children, we have the same night terrors they do, the same horror at having to kiss a decaying old relative, the same sense of helplessness while watching a cherished pet die. Is it, then, so unusual that these equally human individuals, who are only different in that they have had a medical education grafted onto them, respond to patients' fears, and pain, and death in a way that fits in with their own emotional range and their very special temperament?

Some patients are content with a tight-lipped, uncommunicative doctor. Others need the constant feedback of a talkative, bubbly, extroverted one. And then there are the many who are satisfied with someone who is halfway between the two extremes. I am not at all sure what pushed me into having a very verbal and physically demonstrative relationship with my patients and into having an office setup that gave high visibility to my person and my temperament. At the same time, I chose a doctor for myself who was my complete opposite. George did not really ever have very much to say and almost always looked grim when he was examining me or, with agonizing slowness, checking my electrocardiogram, until he finally squeezed out the news that "everything is okay." I often thought about why George was the way he was. I knew that he had had a frightening childhood in wartime Poland, but then again, Marcel, one of our most charming and cheerful colleagues, had been shifted from camp to camp during the same time, lying on top of a freight car and trying to protect his father from the cold of midwinter. And what was the origin of the cult of personality that characterized my practice? Was I really so outgoing, or was I trying to model myself on my father, with his famously warm attitude toward his patients and the casual way in which he ran his office? But whatever the reasons for appearing to our patients the way we did (and they were obviously much more complicated than I have suggested), both George and I were stuck with our temperaments, which had been permanently frozen into place at some unknown time in the past. Did my choice of George as my doctor mean that I preferred his approach to patients over my own? Not at all. It just meant that I respected his medical skills, that I had confidence in him, and that in exchange for this, I was willing to accept his personality quirks, which were not that significant if one compared them, for instance, to Jeff's major behavior disturbance. I am sure, at the same time, that I rubbed some of my own patients the wrong way at one time or another but that they chose to stay with me, probably because of what they perceived as my capabilities and despite some of my own personality quirks.

But the situation becomes even more complicated. If, as many of us do, we first meet our doctor when we are relatively well and find that his temperament is at least acceptable to us, how do we know what is going to happen when the ante is raised—in other words, when we get good and sick? Is the deliberate, quiet one going to be able to raise the emotional energy required when matters become worse, then better, then worse again, let us say, and where much will depend upon his imagination and, most of all, his courage? And, in the same situation, how about the one like me, who may appear a little slick when things are going well, as he is constantly flying goodwill missions around his office? Can he be expected to drop the charm down a few degrees and be trusted to concentrate soberly when a serious clinical problem arises?

I do not pretend to know the answers to these questions, except as they applied to George and to me. When I became acutely ill, George was absolutely tireless in taking extremely solicitous care of me. I say this not as a professional judgment but, much more important, as a patient who felt that he had a caring and effective doctor, though one who was not more verbal than before. And what about me? How did I react when things got tough? Insecurity, uncertainty, and potential guilt, which are unavoidable when we deal with critical illness, had a way of bringing out the best in me and, justifiably, stimulated my efforts way beyond the level of everyday, conscientious medical care. As far as my temperament was concerned, though, I also did not change my spots, as uncertainty, if anything, made me even more talkative and oversolicitous than ever.

I am, of course, only using George and myself as examples. Many doctors, whose temperaments bridge the gap between George's and mine, treat severely ill patients perfectly well. It is just that I don't know how to tell how the individual doctor is going to respond to crisis and whether his very special view of the world, admittedly in a minimum of instances, can keep him from responding adequately.

But there is another dilemma, and that is that the patient's emotional requirements may change drastically during a severe illness. The doctor you choose when you are well may not fit the bill when you are sick. Although, when you were well, you were perfectly satisfied with the sparse facts the quiet doctor doled out to you, now that you are sick you may well be insatiable for detailed information and, more important, reassurance. At the other extreme, you appreciated the warmth and protection the gabby and frequent-cheek-kissing doctor gave you when you were well. But now that you are sick, he may drive you crazy when all you want to do, in your misery, is not to be talked and cuddled to death.

I emphasize all these possible combinations in the feelings of both patients and doctors because they form part of an old problem, and it is this: HOW DO YOU FIND THE RIGHT DOCTOR? Unfortunately, this is a question that, though vitally important, does not have a satisfactory (or even a ready) answer. There is no question about it, there are wild swings in competence among individual doctors. The training and licensing processes assure only minimum capabilities, and beyond that it is often frustrating and confusing for a patient to find someone whose knowledge he can trust. Yet in most communities of our country, a competent doctor can be found. Word of mouth is very important in this search, since patients often have excellent instincts about doctors' skills.

But competence is not all. From firsthand experience, other patients can fill you in on how the doctor runs his practice. Does he understand that you also have a tight schedule and cannot routinely be kept waiting for hours at a time? And how is his staff? Do his assistants treat you respectfully like an adult, or are they either hostile and impatient or, worse yet, over-friendly and prone to immediately calling you by your first name?

Certainly, hospital affiliations, board certification, evidence of good training, and the like help to identify the interested and capable physician. Occasionally, a subpar doctor slips through these safeguards meant to protect the patient. In general, though, a doctor with a reputation for providing conscientious care, and whose qualifications show that he keeps up with recent developments in medicine, is a good bet, as far as competence is concerned, for the prospective patient.

But finding a *good* doctor does not necessarily mean that you have found the *right* doctor. In other words, whether you will connect with the doctor emotionally is completely unpredictable. I wish that interviewing the doctor before actually becoming his patient, something surprisingly few people actually do, were helpful. These preliminary meetings don't usually make any difference, though, because everyone is on his best behavior. Both doctor and patient can afford to be genial. After all, none of the unreasonable, hostile, and demanding traits sometimes artificially produced by sickness are on the table, at least for the time being.

Speaking realistically, there is no way of foreseeing whether you and the doctor who has been recommended to you or to whom you have come by chance will be compatible. Forecasting the success or failure of a marriage on the basis of the personality traits of the principals is known to be very hazardous. There are all kinds of myths, including "opposites attract," "quiet people get along well," and so on. Yet the divorce courts disenchant us daily from these fancies, so that, at bottom, we are no wiser in this area than we ever were. In medicine, just as in marriage, people can be brought together, but that does not mean that they will stay together. Sometimes I arrange a successful match, as when I referred my calm English patient Ruth Herman for surgery to Rob, her emotional counterpart, but it was quite possible that what seemed like a logical plan could have backfired. Experts speak of "chemistry" in trying to explain the merging of two peoples' temperaments into a successful union. But I have studied chemistry, and I have always been under the impression that it is an exact, predictable science—in other words, the exact opposite of the "chemistry" invoked by the romantics. There is something largely irrational connected with why people do or do not get along, so I never know in advance whether my patient and I or my patient and a consultant will hit it off.

At this point, though, I become the romantic because I am convinced that, in medicine as well as in love, there is someone for everyone. Yet the search, again as in love, can be difficult, so a patient may well have to try several doctors before he finds someone with whom he is truly comfortable.

But whether you like your doctor or not should not be considered just some capricious thing that patients have dreamed up. Trust, or faith, in a doctor has something mystical about it, and it can give a large boost to whatever he is doing for you. There is much talk nowadays, and I hope it will soon be reflected in real action, about providing the best possible medical care to all Americans, including those who up to now have had to press their noses against this particular window because of their lack of adequate insurance. When I read about supermarkets with names like "cost containment," or "managed care," or "health care industry," I cannot help but feel a little frightened about what is going to happen to that mom-and-pop store that is not nearly ready to close its doors though it has taken quite a battering all these years, and that is the good old relationship between you and us. I do not doubt that all our citizens will have access to competent medical care in the future, but with all the emphasis on economics and on management and on cost effectiveness (completely justified, by the way), will there be provisions made for universal access to an emotionally satisfying relationship with a doctor?

Tests are inanimate procedures recorded on the by-products of dead trees, x-rays are only pictures of the insides of human beings, and our much beloved "screening" for disease attempts to transform people into cars going down an assembly line. The things that are truly alive in medicine are only the patient, the doctor, and the dynamic link between them. To reduce this link to a mathematical formula, to replace skin-to-skin contact with intermediaries made of metal or film in order to save money or time or (worst of all) bother, is to deny the great tradition of one human being going to the edge to pull another one back from the brink.

Save money? Sure!

Make availability of health care fairer? Absolutely!

Assign a cipher from the army of patients to a random number from the army of doctors? No, no, a thousand times no!

Printed in the United States
By Bookmasters